Medicare

The truth about Medicare & what you should know

1st Edition

Written By:

Kris Keush

Contents

Chapter 1:

Understanding Medicare – Exploring the Inner Workings of Medicare

Addressing Initial Concerns about Medicare 1
Addressing Concerns about Health Issues and Pre-existing Conditions 2
Understanding Costs and Coverage in Medicare 2
Clarifying Coverage Limits and Open Enrollment 3
Enrollment in Medicare and Family Coverage 3
Age and Medicare Coverage 3
Details of the ABC (and D) of Medicare 4
Part A: 4
Part B: 4
Part C: 4
Part D: 5

Chapter 2:

What Medicare Covers

Specialized Care in Special Circumstances 10
Skilled Nursing Facility 10
Home Health Care 11
Hospice Care 11

Medical Supplies - Equipment 13

What Part D Covers: 14

About Formularies 16

Drugs Part D Plans Must Cover 17

Drugs Medicare Doesn't Pay For 17

When Drugs are Covered by Part A, Part B, Part D 17

What Medicare Doesn't Cover 18

Medicare Does Not Cover Safety Items 18

Enrolled in A Medicare Advantage (MA – Plan) 18

Skilled Nursing Facility Has Limits 19

Mental Health Benefits Limits 19

Psychiatric Services – Outpatient 19

In Hospital Psychiatric Care 19

Mental Health Benefits - Medicare Advantage 20

Therapy Services – Limits 20

Co-Payments – Deductibles 20

Limits on Out-of-Pocket 20

D Cost of Part D 20

Enrolled in a Medicare Advantage (MA) Plan 21

Skilled Nursing Facility (SNF) has Limits 21

Mental Health Benefits Limits 21

Psychiatric Services - Outpatient 21

In Hospital Psychiatric Care 21

Mental Health Benefits - Medicare Advantage 22

Therapy Services - Limits 22

Co-Payments and Deductibles 22

Limits on Out-of-Pocket Costs 22

Cost of Part D 22

Chapter 3:

Your Costs in Medicare

Understanding the Costs of Medicare 24

Premiums, Deductibles, and Co-payments 24

Costs Associated with Part A 26

Premiums 26

Deductible 26

Co-payments (hospital-skilled nursing facility) 26

Co-payments (Home Health Care - Hospice Care) 27

Out-of-Pocket Limits 27

Costs Associated with Part B 27

Premiums 27

Costs Associated with Part D 27

Premiums 28

Co-payments 28

Medicare Advantage Costs 28

Deductible 28

Co-payments 29

Out-Of-Pocket Limits 29

Income-Related Premium Surcharge 29

Surcharges Waived 33

Other Situations Qualify for a Waiver 34

Paying Different Premiums 35

Paying Medicare Taxes While Receiving Medicare Benefits: 36

Chapter 4:

Reducing Your Out-of-Pocket Expenses

Exploring Medigap Insurance Options 37

Key Facts about Medigap 37

Understanding Medigap Policies 38

Having a Medigap Policy, That's No Longer Sold 39

Choosing and Buying a Medigap Policy 40

Qualifying for State Assistance 40

Medicaid 40

Medicare Savings Programs 41

What if Social Security Denies My Application? 45

Here are some things to consider when selecting a drug plan: 47

Using Mail Order or Preferred Pharmacies 49

Finding Free or Low-Cost Prescription Drugs 49

Part 2 - The How's and When's of Medicare 49

Eligibility for Medicare 49

Chapter 5:

Qualifying for Medicare

Hitting the Milestone of Age 65 52

Debunking some qualification myths 53

Part A 54

Part B 54

Part C 55

Qualifying for Part A on your own work record 55

Being eligible for Part A on someone else's work record 56

Your spouse, current or past, has sufficient credit 56

Neither you nor your spouse has 40 work credits 57

You're the foreign spouse of a U.S. citizen or legal resident 57

You're in a same sex marriage 57

You are unmarried but live in a domestic partnership 58

Qualifying for Medicare under Age 65 on the Basis of Disability 58

Receiving disability payments 58

How does the 24-month waiting period work? 59

How long does Medicare coverage last? 60

Does railroad retirement disability work in the same way? 60

Suffering from permanent kidney failure (ESRD) 61

Falling through the Cracks: Health-Care Options if You Can't Get Medicare Yet 61

Paying for COBRA temporary insurance 62

Chapter 6:

How to Enroll in Medicare and What to Expect

Having Your Medicare Parts A and B Enrollment Handled Automatically 66

Count Me In! Procedures for Obtaining Medicare Parts A and B 67

To Register Within the United States 67

Signing Up when you are Overseas 67

Retirees Moving in Different States All Year 68

Understanding Medicare Application Jargon 69

Medicare Enrolment

How to Sign up if you are Fully Insured for Benefits of Medicare? 70

How to Enroll if There is no Entirely Insured Medicare Benefits? 70

Medicare Enrollment from outside the US 70

How You May Contact SSA by Mail: 71

How to Contact SSA by Phone: 71

Refusing to Participate in Medicare Parts A and B 71

Declining Part A 71

Opting out of part B 72

Disenrolling from Part B 72

Learning When to Decline Medicare Part B Coverage under 65 73

Getting to Know - Not Accepting Medicare Part B Might Be Risky At Any Age 73

Knowing When Your Coverage Begins 74

When you enroll in the first quarter of your Individualized Education Program 75

When you sign up during IEP months four through seven 76

Chapter 7:

Making Sense of Medicare's Many Options

Gaining Perspective: Step One in Finding Your Way Through Medicare 78

Getting to Know the outcomes of your option for a system 79

Factors to consider while deciding between two systems 80

A fundamental restriction on your choice 81

Weighing the two systems 82

Overall costs 82

Premium costs 83

Co-pay costs 83

Cost and benefit stability 84

Care stability 84

Provider choice and care coordination 85

Extra benefits 85

Geographical area 86

Quality measures 86

Recognizing when you may not have a choice 86

Being on your guard against "auto-enrollment" 87

Comparing Medicare Parts A and B and Medicare Advantage 90

Choosing for Traditional Medicare: 90

Looking at Medicare Advantage Plans 92

Health Maintenance Organizations (HMOs) 93

Preferred Provider Organizations (PPOs) 93

Private Fee-for-Service (PFFS) plans 94

Special Needs Plans (SNPs) 95

Medical Savings Account (MSA) plans 96

Learning About the Variations Between Medigap and MA Plans for Medicare Benefits 98

Chapter 8:

Choosing Medicare Advantage

Medicare Advantage Plans Comparison 100

Comparing Medical Benefits between plans 102
Walking through an example 103
Prescription drug coverage 106
Choosing the Medicare Advantage Plan 109
Which providers accept the plans you're considering 109

Chapter 9:

Discovering the Ins and Outs of Specific Medicare Benefits

Examining Part A 113
Being aware of hospital benefit periods 114
Hospital coverage in traditional Medicare 114
Traditional Medicare's Skilled nursing care in 116
Medicare Advantage plans cover hospitals and skilled nursing facilities 117
Remembering the three-day rule 117
Defining observation status 118
Consequences of being in observation status 119
Premature hospital discharge 121
Your rights in a skilled nursing facility 123
Leaving the SNF 123
Doctor of your choice 125
If Medicare refuses to pay, you may still submit a claim 126

Part B 127

Will Medicare will insure your treatment 127

Ambulance services 129

Find out a service's cost in advance 130

Maximizing your coverage 131

Specific About the Service You Want 132

Other Requirements 132

Your Right to Second Opinions 132

Filing a claim with Medicare 133

Doctor does not file a claim 133

Medicare to deny a claim 134

Part D 134

How a plan may restrict your drug coverage 134

Exception with your doctor's Help 136

Prescriptions from the right doctor 137

Grappling with the tier system of co-pays 138

Pricing Tiers? 138

Find out your plan's pricing tiers? 139

Your drugs are suddenly switched to a higher price tier? 139

Doughnut hole 140

Chapter 10:

Changing Your Medicare and Medigap Coverage

Open Enrollment or Disenrollment Switching Coverage 146

Open enrollment period 146

Disenrollment period 147

Advantages of Special Enrollment Periods 148

When you can use SEPs to change plans 148

Moving permanently outside your plan's service area 148

When you move into or leave a nursing home or other long-term-care facility 149

Medicare Advantage and switching to traditional Medicare 150

Dropping Medigap policy and enroll in a Medicare Advantage for the first time 150

Switching to a five-star plan 151

When your plan withdraws service from your area 151

Dropping a Plan (Or Being Dropped) 154

Leaving a plan on your own 154

Getting the dropped from your current plan 155

Stay or Switch to Another Plan for Next Year 156

Switching to a Medicare Advantage 159

Changing your Medigap Policy 160

Consequences of switching Medigap policies 162

Your right to a 30-day free look 164

Chapter 11:

Medicare Misconceptions

You don't need to Reach Full Retirement Age before Signing Up 165

Don't Assume You Don't Qualify for Medicare 166

It's Crucial to Enroll in Part B When You Should 166

You Need Part B 167

Part D – You still need Prescription Drugs 167

Picking the wrong Part D Drug Plan for the Wrong Reasons 167

Confusion of Enrollment Periods 168

Being unable to purchase Medigap with Full Protection in time 168

Not Reading Your Annual Change Notice 168

Being Aware of Your Potential Eligibility for Cost-Reduction Assistance.... 169

Checkoff List

Checkoff List 171

Personal Information, Family History, & Financial Information

Personal Information, Family History, & Financial Information 171

Chapter 1
Understanding Medicare

Exploring the Inner Workings of Medicare

Topics:

- Addressing common concerns associated with Medicare.
- Gaining insight into the various components of Medicare.
- Recognizing the need for timely decision-making and the array of choices available.

With over 60 million beneficiaries, Medicare is a crucial healthcare expense coverage program for seniors and individuals with disabilities in the United States. Unlike other insurance programs, Medicare is a distinctive national healthcare initiative that extends its benefits to individuals regardless of income, health status, or geographic location. Since its establishment in 1966, Medicare has maintained its popularity among Americans. Nevertheless, it operates on a distinct set of principles and regulations, necessitating a fundamental understanding of its structure to avoid confusion.

This chapter provides an overarching view of Medicare, outlining its unique features compared to other health insurance options. Additionally, it explores the four coverage parts of Medicare (A, B, C, and D). It presents a decision-making checklist to help navigate the selection of coverage options offered by the program. The information presented here is tailored for individuals new to Medicare seeking essential knowledge about the program.

Addressing Initial Concerns about Medicare

As individuals approach the possibility of becoming Medicare beneficiaries, many find themselves realizing their limited understanding of the program. Doubts may arise regarding the accuracy of the information available, particularly in light of the prevalence of misconceptions perpetuated through mass emails or misleading internet sources. If you have had previous health insurance, especially through an employer, you might feel apprehensive about how Medicare coverage compares to your prior plan.

One common concern is whether Medicare, as a government-run system, will provide subpar care. The answer is no, or at least not inherently. Although the federal government administers and oversees Medicare, with most medical services being federally funded, the actual provision of these services primarily falls under the purview of private entities. The doctors you see are not government employees, and the hospitals and laboratories that render their services are not government-owned. These private entities have the freedom to decide whether or not to enter into contracts with Medicare. The independent practitioners who accept Medicare patients are the same private doctors you would have consulted for diagnosis and treatment before enrolling in Medicare.

Another concern often raised is whether Medicare will restrict one's choices. Contrary to this concern, Medicare offers an extensive range of options and expands one's choices in some instances. If you previously had health insurance through a private employer, you likely had limited plan options each year. In contrast, Medicare provides a choice between the traditional program, which allows you to see any doctor or provider in the US accepting Medicare patients and various private Medicare Advantage health plans that resemble plans you may have had in the past.

Depending on your location, you may have many options, with specific areas offering up to 28 Medicare Advantage plans. Furthermore, each state provides up to 50 Part D plans, delivering Medicare prescription drug coverage. The subsequent section will delve into the details of Medicare Advantage and Part D plans, highlighting their distinctions from the traditional program.

Addressing Concerns about Health Issues and Pre-existing Conditions

Another prevalent concern among individuals is whether their health issues or pre-existing medical conditions will affect their Medicare coverage or result in higher premiums or co-pays. The answer is no, as Medicare does not discriminate based on current or past health problems. Unlike private health insurance, Medicare does not impose higher rates or deny coverage due to pre-existing conditions. There is only one exception—individuals with advanced kidney failure cannot enroll in a Medicare Advantage health plan. Nevertheless, under the traditional Medicare program, they can still receive coverage for necessary care, such as regular dialysis or a kidney transplant. It is also worth noting that a history of smoking, alcohol use, or obesity does not impact Medicare rates.

Understanding Costs and Coverage in Medicare

To summarize, Medicare is not free and requires the payment of monthly premiums, deductibles, and co-pays. However, when compared to most employer insurance, Medicare is reasonably priced. Without Medicare, many older and disabled individuals would struggle to find affordable insurance in the open market. In 2020, monthly premiums for Medicare Part B were $144.60 per person. In contrast, workers' monthly contributions to employer insurance averaged $99 for a single person and $462 for a family of two or more, according to the Kaiser Family Foundation's 2019 survey of employer health benefits.

It is important to note that this comparison is not exact, as many employees pay more than these averages for health benefits. Additionally, Medicare beneficiaries usually pay extra for drug coverage, and individuals with higher incomes may have higher Part B premiums than the standard rates.

While Medicare has deductibles, they tend to be smaller than those in high-deductible health plans provided by employers or obtained through the Affordable Care Act or the open insurance market.

Clarifying Coverage Limits and Open Enrollment

The traditional Medicare program has no out-of-pocket spending limit or cap on the costs that beneficiaries may incur for their healthcare services each year. However, as mentioned earlier, beneficiaries can purchase Medigap insurance to cover these costs. On the other hand, all Medicare Advantage plans are legally required to establish a limit on out-of-pocket expenses, which can vary depending on the specific strategy.

Similarly, in the Part D program, there is a coverage gap, often called the "donut hole," where beneficiaries pay a higher percentage of their prescription drug fees until they reach the catastrophic coverage point, significantly lowering their costs for the remainder of the year.

Enrollment in Medicare and Family Coverage

Enrollment in Medicare does not need to occur every year. Coverage automatically continues year after year unless changes are desired. However, there is an open enrollment period from October 15 to December 7 each year, during which individuals can change their coverage if desired. This includes switching from traditional Medicare to a Medicare Advantage plan, changing from one Medicare Advantage plan to another, or switching from one Part D prescription drug plan to another.

It is important to note that Medicare does not offer family coverage for spouses, dependent children, or other family members. Each individual must wait until age 65 to join the program unless they qualify through disability at a younger age.

Moreover, if both spouses are enrolled in Medicare, they must pay separate and total premiums unless they receive government assistance to help cover the costs.

Age and Medicare Coverage

Medicare coverage is not based on age but rather on medical necessity. Therefore, even if you require a medical procedure such as a hip replacement in your 90s or over 100, Medicare will still cover most of the cost, just as it would for anyone else.

The notion that Medicare limits care and denies coverage based on age has been disseminated through mass emails to discredit the Affordable Care Act. However, no Medicare regulations restrict care for individuals based on age, and the Act does not reduce Medicare benefits or permit rationing.

Details of the ABC (and D) of Medicare

Understanding the details of what Parts A, B, C, and D stand for is crucial for comprehending how Medicare functions. Each component of Medicare determines the coverage you receive and the costs you incur. Here is a breakdown of each Part:

Part A:

Part A is often called "hospital insurance," but it covers more than just inpatient hospital stays. It also includes coverage for services provided in settings beyond the hospital, such as nursing care.

Coverage under Part A includes services like professional nursing care during hospital stays or stays in skilled nursing facilities, semiprivate rooms, meals, and other services provided directly by hospitals or nursing facilities. Part A also covers home health services and hospice care.

Many Medicare beneficiaries do not have to pay premiums for Part A services since Medicare payroll taxes fund it. However, deductibles and co-payments still apply for certain services.

Part B:

Part B, known as medical insurance, covers many services that most Medicare beneficiaries will eventually need, even if they never require hospitalization. Services covered by Part B include medical and surgical services from doctors who accept Medicare patients, diagnostic and lab tests outside of hospitals, preventive services, medical equipment and supplies, outpatient hospital treatment, and more.

Part B requires a monthly premium unless the individual qualifies for state assistance due to low income. The standard premium in 2020 was $144.60. Beneficiaries are responsible for a percentage of the cost of most Part B services, typically 20% of the Medicare-approved price under traditional Medicare. Medicare Advantage plans may have different cost-sharing structures.

Part C:

Part C, also known as Medicare Advantage, offers an alternative to traditional Medicare. It provides managed care through Health Maintenance Organizations (HMOs) or Preferred Provider Organizations (PPOs) administered by private insurance companies. Medicare Advantage plans receive a fixed fee from Medicare for each plan member, regardless of the amount of healthcare they use. These plans must offer the same services that Part A and Part B cover, with additional benefits like routine dental, hearing, and vision care and Part D prescription drug coverage.

There are differences between traditional Medicare and Medicare Advantage plans regarding out-of-pocket costs and provider options.

Part D:

Part D is the prescription drug coverage component of Medicare. It helps beneficiaries pay for prescription medications. Private insurance companies approved by Medicare offer Part D plans. These plans have a formulary, a list of covered drugs and may have different tiers and cost-sharing structures. Beneficiaries pay a monthly premium, a deductible, and a portion of the drug costs until they reach the catastrophic coverage threshold, where their costs decrease significantly.

Understanding Medicare's ABC (and D) is essential for navigating the program and making informed decisions about coverage and healthcare options. A monthly premium is required to access Part B services unless the individual qualifies for state assistance due to low income. The standard Part B premium is determined annually by a formula established by law, which was $144.60 in 2020. If the individual's income exceeds a certain level, they may be charged more.

In addition to the monthly premium, beneficiaries are responsible for a percentage of the cost of most Part B services. Under traditional Medicare, this is typically 20% of the Medicare-approved cost. However, Medicare Advantage plans charge varying amounts, usually fixed-dollar co-pays, for each service. Part C, also known as Medicare Advantage, provides an alternative to traditional Medicare. The coverage provided by Part A and Part B is collectively known as traditional or original Medicare. It is referred to as fee-for-service Medicare because providers are paid a fee for each service they provide.

Medicare Advantage plans, on the other hand, provide managed care through Health Maintenance Organizations (HMOs) or Preferred Provider Organizations (PPOs) administered by private insurance companies. Medicare Advantage plans receive a fixed fee from Medicare for each plan member, regardless of the amount of healthcare they use. These plans are required by law to offer the same services covered by Part A and Part B as traditional Medicare, including procedures like knee replacements. Medicare Advantage plans may also provide additional benefits not covered by traditional Medicare, such as routine dental, hearing, and vision care and Part D prescription drug coverage. However, there are differences between traditional Medicare and Medicare Advantage plans regarding out-of-pocket costs and provider options.

Part D is a form of insurance that covers the cost of outpatient prescription drugs. It was introduced to Medicare in 2006, and it helps individuals save money on medications and access drugs they may not have been able to afford previously. However, navigating Part D can be complex.

Here are some key points to consider:

- Coverage is divided into four phases throughout the year, and the cost of drugs can vary between these phases.

- Beneficiaries must choose only one private plan from the available options (at least 15) that provide Part D drugs.
- Various plans cover different sets of drugs, and no plan encircles all drugs. Co-pays for each drug can vary widely between plans.
- Plans may require prior authorization for certain drugs or need individuals to try a less-expensive version first.
- Plans can change costs and benefits or even withdraw from Medicare yearly.

Despite the complexity, there are strategies for comparing plans and finding the best coverage for individual needs. It's important to carefully review plan details, including drug formularies, co-pays, and coverage restrictions or requirements. Regarding Medicare, some choices and decisions must be made within specific timeframes.

To ensure you make informed decisions, consider the following checklist:

- Enroll at the right time to avoid permanent financial penalties and ensure coverage when needed.
- Research your options and understand the differences between traditional Medicare and Medicare Advantage health plans.
- If you opt for traditional Medicare, make smart choices, such as whether to add Part D prescription drug coverage and Medigap supplemental insurance.
- If you opt for a Medicare Advantage plan, compare plans based on your needs and understand your options to switch to traditional Medicare if needed.
- Seek help from legitimate and informed sources to make your choices and avoid scams and fraud.
- Understand your right to change your coverage every year and at other times under certain circumstances.
- Learn about the purpose of various enrollment periods, their deadlines, and the process of switching to another plan or type of coverage.

Making the right choices and understanding the available options will help ensure you have the coverage you need and avoid unnecessary penalties or complications. It's important to stay informed and utilize the resources available to help you navigate the Medicare system.

Chapter 2
What Medicare Covers

Topics:

- Understanding the scope of coverage provided by Medicare Part A and Part B
- Understanding the coverage provided by Medicare Part D
- Being aware of what is not covered by Medicare.
- Understanding that some types of coverage have limits or restrictions.

However, when it comes to receiving these services at no cost, it's important to understand that you need to visit a doctor who accepts the Medicare-approved amount as payment in full for any service provided to a Medicare patient. This is commonly referred to as accepting assignment. If a doctor does not accept assignment, you may be required to pay a co-pay or even the full cost of the service.

Table 2-1 provides a comprehensive range of preventive tests, screenings, and counseling sessions covered under Medicare Part B. It also indicates whether there is any cost associated with each service. This table showcases the impressive array of covered services available to Medicare beneficiaries.

It's essential to be aware of the providers who accept assignments in order to take advantage of the no-cost coverage for these preventive services. By visiting Medicare-approved doctors and healthcare professionals, you can receive the necessary screenings, tests, and counseling without incurring additional expenses.

TABLE 2-1 Preventive Care Services Medicare Covers

Service	Frequency Covered	Cost to You
"Welcome to Medicare"	Once only, during first	Free, but any other
checkup	12 months in Part B.	tests the doctor refers you for may require a co-pay.
Wellness checkup	Once every 12 months, after you've had Part B for one year.	Free as long as you ask for a wellness visit and not a "Physical."
Abdominal aortic	One-time ultrasound	Free.

aneurysm screening	for people at risk.	
Alcohol misuse screening and counseling	One screening and up to four counseling sessions a year.	Free.
Bone mass measurements	Once a year If you're at risk for broken bones; more if medically necessary	Free.
Breast cancer screening (mammograms)	Once a year for women age 40 or older.	Free.
Cardiovascular disease (Behavioral therapy)	Once a year.	Free.
Cardiovascular disease screening	Once every five years.	Free for the tests, but a co-pay is usually required for the doctor visit.
Cervical/vaginal cancer screening	Once every 24 months, or every 12 months if you're at high risk.	Free.
Colorectal cancer screening - barium enema when used instead of flexible sigmoidoscopy or colonoscopy)	Once every 48 months, or every 24 months if at high risk	A co-pay is required.
Colorectal cancer screening - colonoscopy	Once every 120 months, or every 24 months if at high risk.	Free for the test, but a co-pay is required if a polyp is found and removed during the test.
Colorectal cancer screening - fecal occult blood test	Once every 12 months if you're 50 or older.	Free.

Colorectal cancer screening - flexible sigmoidoscopy	Once every 48 months if you're 50 or older.	Free.
Depression screening	Once a year in a primary-care setting.	Free screening, but a co-pay is required for doctor visit and follow-up care.
Diabetes training	Training on how to self-manage diabetes - up to 12 hours in the first year and up to two hours every year after that.	A co-pay is required, and your Part B deductible applies
Diabetes screening	Up to two screenings a year if you're at risk of developing diabetes.	Free.
Flu shots	Once a year in flu season.	Free.
Glaucoma (eye disease Tests	Once every 12 months if you're at high risk.	A co-pay is required, and your Part B deductible applies.
Hepatitis B virus (HPV) infection screening	Annually only for those considered at risk who doesn't get a Hepatitis B vaccination.	Free.
Hepatitis C screening test	One-time screening; yearly screening for people at high risk or those born between 1945 and 1965.	Free.
HIV screenings	Once every 12 months or up to three times during pregnancy.	Free.
Lung cancer screening	Once a year for people age 55-77, who are current or former smokers averaging one pack a day for 30 years, but without symptoms of lung disease.	Free.

Obesity screening and counseling	Behavioral counseling sessions if your body mass index BMI) is 30	Free.
	Or higher	
Pneumococcal shot	After age 65, one type of shot followed at least one year later by a second shot.	Free
Prostate cancer digital rectal exam	Once every 12 months for men over 50.	A co-pay is required, and the Part B deductible applies
Prostate cancer PSA test	Once every 12 months for men over 50.	Free
Sexually transmitted infections screenings and counseling	Tests once every 12 months or more often if pregnant. Up to two counseling sessions with a primary-care provider	Free if tests are ordered by a doctor and performed in a Medicare-approved laboratory.
Smoking and tobacco use cessation counseling	Up to eight sessions in any 12-month period.	Free
X-rays, MRIs, CT scans, EKGs, and so on	As ordered by a doctor and performed in a Medicare	A co-pay is required, and your Part B deductible applies.

Specialized Care in Special Circumstances

Medicare provides specialized care through different parts of the program. Medicare Part A focuses on inpatient hospital care and some technical services outside the hospital, particularly nursing care. On the other hand, Medicare Part B covers a broad range of specialized care, including outpatient services like physical therapy.

Skilled Nursing Facility

Suppose you need specialized nursing care after being discharged from a hospital. In that case, Medicare Part A covers the cost of your ongoing care at a skilled nursing facility, often a nursing home.

However, certain conditions must be met to qualify for this coverage. You're formally admitted to a hospital for at least three days, and a doctor must prescribe the necessary services provided by qualified professionals such as registered nurses and physical or speech therapists. Additionally, the skilled nursing facility you choose must be approved by

Medicare. Under traditional Medicare, you can receive coverage for stays at a skilled nursing facility for up to 100 days within a benefit period.

The first 20 days are covered at no cost to you. From day 21 to day 100, you are responsible for a daily co-pay, which slightly increases yearly (e.g., in 2020, it was $176 per day). However, some Medigap supplemental insurance policies fully cover these co-pays. If you have a Medicare Advantage health plan, you should review your coverage documents or contact your plan to determine the cost of staying in skilled nursing facilities.

Home Health Care

Medicare offers home health care services that bring skilled nursing and therapy care to your home, providing similar care to what you would receive in a skilled nursing facility. These services include part-time skilled nursing care, physical, speech, and occupational therapy, home health aide assistance, medical supplies, and medical social services.

To qualify for Medicare coverage, you need to meet certain criteria. You must be homebound, meaning it is difficult to leave your home without assistance or not recommended for your health. You must also have a doctor's certification of need and be under a doctor's plan of care. Additionally, you must receive care from a Medicare-approved home health agency.

The home health agency must inform you of the associated cost if you require a service or item that Medicare doesn't cover. If you need medical equipment while receiving home health care, you can obtain it through the agency, but you will be responsible for a 20% co-pay unless you have Medigap insurance that covers the cost.

Hospice Care

Medicare covers hospice care, which focuses on providing comfort and support for individuals in their final days or months of life. It is available to terminally ill patients and their caregivers at minimal cost. Hospice care offers a comprehensive range of medical and support services, often provided in the patient's home, with the option of inpatient care in a hospital or nursing home for respite care.

To qualify for the hospice benefit, you must meet the following conditions:

- Choose comfort-focused hospice care and forgo treatments intended to cure your terminal illness.
- The medical director of a hospice program and your doctor must confirm a probable life expectancy of less than six months.
- Enroll in a Medicare-approved hospice program and have Medicare Part A hospital insurance.

Medicare covers 100% of the costs for several services related to hospice care, including:

- Medical and nursing care
- 24/7 on-call support
- Medical equipment and supplies
- Homemaker and home health care services
- Physical therapy
- Social worker services
- Dietary counseling
- Caregiver support
- Grief and loss counseling

Additional details regarding hospice care coverage:

- The maximum cost for medication used to control symptoms and pain of your terminal illness is $5 per prescription.
- If you need temporary nursing home admission to give your caregiver a break, you will pay 5% of the cost for respite care.
- Medigap supplemental insurance fully covers both medication costs and respite care expenses.
- Medical costs related to any medical condition other than your terminal illness are covered by Medicare Part B or Part D in the usual manner.

You can discontinue hospice care at any point, and if you wish, you can resume it again. Even if you outlive the six-month prognosis, Medicare coverage continues as long as your doctor and the hospice doctor certify that you're terminally ill. The benefit will end if your health improves and the doctors determine that you no longer need hospice care. However, you have the right to contest this decision, and if your health declines again, the user may be reinstated.

Palliative Care

Palliative care aims to alleviate the symptoms of pain and suffering related to a serious illness that may not be terminal but is considered life-threatening. It focuses on enhancing the quality of life for patients and their caregivers. Unlike hospice care, palliative care does not need patients to forego attempts to cure their illnesses. It can be provided at any time, regardless of the patient's life expectancy.

End-of-Life Counseling

End-of-life counseling, also known as advance care planning, is crucial for individuals to devise their preferences for end-of-life care. It ensures their wishes are honored even if they cannot communicate them due to illness. During an end-of-life counseling session, patients may receive information on creating an advance care directive, a legal document outlining their desired medical treatment in the event of incapacity, and designating a person with medical power of attorney. The session may also cover topics related to hospice and palliative care.

Medicare covers these counseling sessions as a voluntary benefit that patients can receive at any point, whether they are healthy or receiving medical care. If necessary, the first 30 minutes and subsequent sessions are covered by Medicare without a limit on the number of sessions. Counseling sessions can be held in various settings, and if conducted during an annual wellness visit, they are free of charge. However, if a separate session is scheduled, patients must pay the usual Part B co-pay and deductible unless they have supplemental insurance.

Pregnancy - Childbirth

Medicare covers pregnancy and childbirth for those who qualify, including younger people who are eligible through disability. Skilled medical management is covered throughout the pregnancy, from diagnosis to delivery and postnatal care. Medicare also covers treatment for miscarriages and abortions in cases of incest, rape, or life-threatening pregnancies, but not elective abortions. Part A coverage is required for hospital services, while doctors' services and outpatient procedures require Part B coverage. Low-income individuals enrolled in Medicaid may have their Medicare out-of-pocket costs covered by Medicaid. Medicaid may also cover medical care for the newborn, but Medicare does not cover any services for the baby after birth.

Medical Supplies - Equipment

Medicare provides coverage for durable medical equipment, which refers to long-lasting items that help you function but are not considered services or treatments. To be eligible for coverage, these items must be medically necessary, prescribed by a doctor or another primary-care professional, not easily used by anyone who isn't unwell or wounded, reusable and likely to last for three years or more, suitable for use within the home, and provided by Medicare-approved suppliers. Medicare Part B covers durable medical equipment such as walkers, crutches, scooters, manual and powered wheelchairs, commode chairs, hospital beds, respiratory assistance devices, pacemakers, prosthetics (such as artificial limbs and eyes), orthotics (such as limb, neck, and back braces), and other items.

Medicare also covers supplies like diabetic test strips and lancets but generally does not cover disposable items like catheters and diapers. Medicare requires a doctor to complete and sign a Certificate of Medical Necessity for coverage for specific durable medical equipment, such as oxygen equipment or seat lifts. It is the responsibility of your doctor and supplier, not you, to provide the necessary proof of eligibility. Medical equipment is typically rented, but some items may be purchased. Use a supplier that accepts the Medicare-approved amount as full payment. Medicare Part B will cover 80% of the cost, and you'll be responsible for the remaining 20% (unless you have Medigap insurance that covers your share). In a Medicare Advantage plan, coverage is the same, but co-pays may differ, and you should consult your plan for specifics.

What Part D Covers:

- Medicare's Part D program covers prescription drugs; understanding its nuances is essential before enrolling.
- Part D coverage has four phases that can affect how you pay for medications throughout the year.
- The number of phases you experience depends on the cost of your prescription drugs and whether you qualify for Extra Help.

Here is a breakdown of the four phases:

Phase 1: Annual deductible, where you pay the total price for drugs until reaching a limit set by law.

Phase 2: Initial coverage period where you pay plan-required co-payments for each prescription, and the plan covers the rest until reaching a dollar limit set by law.

Phase 3: Coverage gap, also known as the "doughnut hole," starting when the initial coverage limit is reached and ending when your out-of-pocket spending on drugs comes another dollar limit set by law.

The coverage gap is gradually shrinking due to the Affordable Care Act. In the coverage gap, your plan covers at least 5% of the cost of covered brand-name drugs, and you receive a 70% discount on brand-name drugs from the manufacturer. In the coverage gap, Medicare covers 75% of the price for generic drugs, so that you would pay only 25% for generic and brand-name drugs.

Phase 4: Catastrophic coverage begins if your drug costs are high enough to close the coverage gap.

During catastrophic coverage, your share of the costs decreases significantly, and you pay no more than 5% of the price of each prescription.

Catastrophic coverage ends on December 31, and the cycle restarts on January 1 with Phase 1 or 2, depending on your plan's deductible.

Figure 2-1 is a quick way of looking at the same cycle of coverage.

Phase of Coverage	What It Means in Each Calendar Year	2019 Limits	2020 Limits

1. Annual Deductible (if your plan has one)	You pay 100% of your drug costs before coverage begins, until you reach your plan's deductible, which must fall under the maximum limit set by law.	$415	$435
2. Initial coverage	You pay a co-pay for each prescription, and your plan pays the rest until these total drug costs reach the limit.	$3,820	$4,020
3. Coverage gap (Doughnut hole)	Your plan provides no coverage, but you receive discounts from the drug makers and the government until your out-of-pocket spending in the year (including most discounts) reaches the limit.	$5,100	$6,350
4. Catastrophic coverage	You pay about 5% and your plan pays 95% of your drug costs.	$7653.75	$9038.75

FIGURE 2-1: Phases of Part D drug coverage and dollar limits.

Figure 2-2 shows this information in a different way. Here, you can see examples of brand-name drugs costing (for the sake of simplicity) $100, $200, or $300 per one-month prescription – and what you'd pay for them in each phase of coverage. These examples assume co-pays during the initial coverage period of $45 for each prescription, although co-pays vary widely among Part D plans.

Phase of Coverage	What You Pay for a Drug Who's Full One Month Cost Is $100	What You Pay for a - Drug Who's Full One Month Cost Is $200	What You Pay for a - Drug Who's Full One Month Cost Is $300
1. Annual deductible (If your plan has one)	$100	$200	$300

2. Initial coverage (with co-pay of $45)	$45	$45	$45
3. Doughnut hole (you pay 25% for brand-name drugs in 2020)	$25	$50	$75
4. Catastrophic coverage (You pay 5%)	$5	$10	$15

FIGURE 2-2: Examples of costs through four phases of coverage.

About Formularies

Understanding the term "formulary" is crucial in Part D because it directly affects the cost of your medications. Simply put, a formulary refers to the list of drugs each Part D plan chooses to cover. There is no national formulary that all plans must follow, so it's essential to ensure that the drugs you need are included in your plan's formulary. If a drug is not covered, you will be responsible for the full cost unless you can obtain an exception from the plan. The difference in out-of-pocket expenses between a covered and uncovered drug can be significant, potentially amounting to hundreds of dollars monthly.

Additionally, drugs not covered by your plan will not count toward the out-of-pocket limit, which is important to consider if you fall into the coverage gap (Phase 3). Coverage for your prescribed medications is crucial for your overall health because it increases the likelihood of taking medications as prescribed and not skipping doses. However, it's important to note that no Part D plan covers all prescription drugs, and the number of drugs covered can vary greatly from one plan to another. According to Avalere Health, in 2019, only 63% of drugs were covered by Medicare Part D plans. Therefore, choosing a plan that covers most, if not all, of the specific drugs you require, is crucial.

Drugs Part D Plans Must Cover

Medicare law does not require Part D plans to cover every drug, but they must cover at least two drugs in each class of medication. A class refers to a group of similar drugs used to treat the same medical condition. Some plans may cover more than two drugs in each class. However, there are six classes of drugs for which every plan must cover "all or substantially all" drugs. These classes are anticancer drugs, anticonvulsants, antidepressants, antipsychotics, HIV/AIDS drugs, and immunosuppressants. Medicare mandates that all Part D plans cover nearly all drugs in these categories to prevent potential clinical issues arising from patients abruptly stopping or changing such medications.

Drugs Medicare Doesn't Pay For

Certain types of drugs are not covered by Medicare by law, although Part D plans are not prohibited from covering them. Medicare does not reimburse the cost of these drugs. While a few plans may cover some of these drugs, most plans do not cover any of them. The excluded drugs include medicines sold over the counter (not needing a doctor's prescription), drugs used for anorexia, weight loss, or weight gain, drugs used for cosmetic reasons and hair growth, drugs used to promote fertility, drugs used to treat sexual or erectile dysfunction, medicines used to treat cough or cold symptoms, and prescription vitamins and mineral products. However, some medications in these categories may be covered by Medicare if deemed medically necessary, such as cough medicines prescribed by a doctor to treat asthma or medications used to address medical conditions that affect veins and arteries. Additionally, as of 2013, Part D plans can cover barbiturates and benzodiazepines for any medically accepted use, although they were previously not covered due to the potential for abuse.

When Drugs are Covered by Part A, Part B, Part D

It can be unclear, but there are instances where medication may be covered under Medicare Part D and either Part A or B. Some drugs were already covered under Part A or Part B before the creation of Part D, and this practice has continued. As a general guideline, Part A covers drugs administered during a hospital stay or in a skilled nursing facility. In contrast, Part B covers drugs administered in a doctor's office, hospital outpatient departments, and sometimes by a hospice or home healthcare professional. Part D, on the other hand, covers outpatient drugs you or your caregiver administer at home or receive while living in a nursing home.

However, some situations can make these general rules more complex. For example, if you had an organ transplant covered by Medicare, the immunosuppressant drugs required after the surgery would be covered under Part B. If Medicare did not cover the transplant surgery itself, then the drugs would be covered under Part D. If a drug is already covered by either Part A or B, Part D will not pay for it. In such cases, your Part D plan may require additional information from you and your doctor, and prior authorization may be necessary to determine whether the drug should be covered by Part A, B, or D.

What Medicare Doesn't Cover

Medicare does not cover routine dental, vision, hearing, or foot care services. This includes services such as dental cleanings and fillings, eye exams for eyeglasses or contact lenses, hearing aids and exams for fitting them, and routine foot care like nail trimming. However, Medicare will cover these services if needed to diagnose or treat a medical condition. For example, if you have diabetes and need foot care to prevent or treat a foot ulcer, Medicare will cover it. Similarly, Medicare will cover exams and treatment if you have an eye disease like glaucoma or cataracts. There are exceptions where coverage may be provided for routine foot care related to medical conditions such as diabetes, cancer, multiple sclerosis, chronic kidney disease, malnutrition, or vein inflammation caused by blood clots. Additionally, suppose toenail clipping risks your health and requires professional attention. In that case, Medicare may provide coverage with evidence from your doctor or podiatrist that such care is medically necessary.

Medicare Does Not Cover Safety Items

While Medicare spends billions of dollars annually on treating the consequences of falls among older Americans, it does not cover safety items that help prevent falls. Although it covers a few items considered medically reasonable if a doctor prescribes, such as seat lifts or trapeze bars, Medicare does not cover items it deems for convenience rather than medical necessity. Non-covered items include stair lifts or elevators, bathtub lifts or seats, grab bars, room heaters, air conditioners, humidifiers, posture chairs, massage devices, physical fitness equipment, and medical emergency alert systems. However, there are other ways to seek assistance. Disabled veterans can take advantage of programs the Department of Veterans Affairs provides, which offer cash grants to help eligible veterans make safety improvements in their homes. Another option is contacting the non-profit organization Rebuilding Together, which provides volunteers to make housing repairs and install safety equipment free of charge.

Additionally, if you file itemized tax returns, you can deduct the costs of home improvements made for medical reasons.

Enrolled in A Medicare Advantage (MA – Plan)

The payment system for hospital stays under Medicare Advantage plans is typically more straightforward than traditional Medicare. Many plans charge a daily co-pay for the initial days, and then there's no charge for the remaining days. Unlike traditional Medicare, most Medicare Advantage plans don't have a cap on the number of covered days, so you don't need to use lifetime reserve days.

However, some Medicare Advantage plans to cap the number of days covered, although they may not require co-pays for lifetime reserve days. Understanding the differences between traditional Medicare and Medicare Advantage plans regarding hospital stays is crucial.

Skilled Nursing Facility Has Limits

If you require skilled nursing care after a hospital stay and satisfy specific conditions, Medicare provides coverage for a stay in a skilled nursing facility, but it has limitations. For each benefit period, Medicare will cover 100 days of skilled nursing care, and you'll be responsible for the entire cost beyond that.

However, some or all these costs may be covered if you have additional insurance, such as Medicaid, employer health benefits, long-term-care insurance, or Medigap supplemental insurance. It is recommended to check your policy to determine the coverage. Medicare Advantage plans also have restrictions; coverage is usually limited to 100 days in a benefit period.

Mental Health Benefits Limits

Like many other insurance plans, Medicare has traditionally treated mental health care differently than other health issues. While this kind of discrimination is less prevalent in Medicare today, some restrictions remain on mental health benefits, which will be explained in the following sections.

Psychiatric Services – Outpatient

Historically, Medicare treated mental health care differently than other medical care, imposing higher co-pays on outpatient visits to mental health professionals. This disparity has since decreased due to a law passed in 2008, which resulted in reduced co-payments for outpatient psychiatric care. Today, patients must pay the standard 20 percent co-pay for outpatient psychiatric care, and Medicare covers the remainder, provided they see a participating provider. Medigap insurance plans typically cover these co-pays, while those enrolled in Medicare Advantage must pay according to their plan requirements.

In Hospital Psychiatric Care

The healthcare law passed in 2008 did not address discrimination in Medicare policy that limits patients to 190 days of inpatient treatment in psychiatric hospitals over their lifetime. In contrast, there is no such limit for general hospitals. Any days spent in a non-psychiatric hospital, even if the patient is being treated for a mental health condition, will not count towards the 190-day limit.

Medicare covers partial hospitalization in certain situations, including receiving mental health treatment during the day at a hospital's outpatient department, clinic, or community mental health center, without spending the night there. The costs for this type of service depend on the treatment provided, but it can be at most 40 percent of the Medicare-approved amount. However, Part B deductible and co-insurance apply to partial hospitalization services.

Mental Health Benefits - Medicare Advantage

To ensure you clearly understand your mental health benefits under a Medicare Advantage plan, reviewing the plan's evidence of coverage documents is important. While some plans may vary in their coverage for mental health benefits, most Medicare Advantage plans typically adhere to the same 190-day lifetime limit for inpatient care in a psychiatric hospital.

Therapy Services – Limits

Medicare Part B covers physical therapy, speech-language pathology, and occupational therapy. Previously, there was a limit on the amount of coverage for therapy services in any given year, known as the therapy cap. However, as of 2019, Medicare removed the cap and now covers outpatient therapy at 80 percent of the Medicare-approved amount.

If you see a participating provider, you will be responsible for a 20 percent co-pay after meeting the Part B deductible of $198 in 2020. These limits represent the total cost of the services received in a year, including what Medicare and you pay. If you require ongoing therapy for conditions such as stroke or heart disease, Medicare may cover these services beyond the annual limits if your therapist justifies the need. Medicare automatically reviews your case if the total cost reaches $3,000 in a year.

Co-Payments – Deductibles

The Part B deductible in 2020 amounted to $198 and is typically adjusted slightly higher each year, with the new amount announced alongside the Part B premium. Generally, Medicare covers 80 percent of the Medicare-approved cost for Part B services, and you are responsible for the remaining 20 percent. However, if you receive care from a provider who does not accept the Medicare-approved cost as full payment, you may be charged more than 20 percent.

Limits on Out-of-Pocket

Under traditional Medicare, Part B has no maximum cap on out-of-pocket expenses. However, if you have Medigap supplemental insurance, your Part B co-pays will be fully or partially covered based on the policy you purchase.

D Cost of Part D

Part D covers prescription drugs prescribed by a doctor and taken by the patient at home. To access this coverage, you can enroll in a standalone Part D drug plan if you have traditional Medicare for your medical benefits. Alternatively, you can opt for a Medicare Advantage plan with medical and Part D drug coverage within its benefits package.

Enrolled in a Medicare Advantage (MA) Plan

When enrolled in a Medicare Advantage (MA) plan, the payment system for hospital stays is typically more straightforward than traditional Medicare. Most MA plans charge a daily co-pay for the initial days of a hospital stay, and there may be no charge for the remaining days. Unlike traditional Medicare, most MA plans do not cap the number of covered days, so there is no need to use lifetime reserve days.

However, it's important to note that some Medicare Advantage plans may cap the number of days covered, although they may not require co-pays for lifetime reserve days. Understanding the differences between traditional Medicare and Medicare Advantage plans regarding hospital stays is crucial to making informed healthcare decisions.

Skilled Nursing Facility (SNF) has Limits

If you require skilled nursing care after a hospital stay and meet specific conditions, Medicare provides coverage for a stay in a skilled nursing facility. However, there are limitations to this coverage. Medicare will cover 100 days of professional nursing care for each benefit period. Beyond that, you will be responsible for the entire cost.

Some or all of these costs may be covered if you have additional insurance, such as Medicaid, employer health benefits, long-term care insurance, or a Medigap supplemental insurance policy. It's essential to check your policy to determine the extent of coverage. Medicare Advantage plans also have restrictions; coverage is usually limited to 100 days in a benefit period.

Mental Health Benefits Limits

Medicare has traditionally treated mental health care differently than other health issues, but the disparities have decreased. However, there are still some restrictions on mental health benefits under Medicare.

Psychiatric Services - Outpatient

Medicare covers outpatient psychiatric care, and the co-pays for these visits have been reduced due to a law passed in 2008. Patients must typically pay the standard 20% co-pay for outpatient psychiatric care, and Medicare covers the remainder, provided they see a participating provider. Medigap insurance plans often cover these co-pays, while those enrolled in Medicare Advantage must pay according to their plan's requirements.

In Hospital Psychiatric Care

Medicare sets a limit of 190 days of inpatient treatment in psychiatric hospitals over a lifetime, whereas there is no such limit for general hospitals. Any days spent in a non-psychiatric hospital, even if the patient is being treated for a mental health condition, will not count towards the 190-day limit.

Medicare covers partial hospitalization in certain situations, which involves receiving mental health treatment during the day at a hospital's outpatient department, clinic, or community mental health center, without spending the night there. The costs for this type of service depend on the treatment provided but can be at most 40% of the Medicare-approved amount. However, Part B deductible and co-insurance apply to partial hospitalization services.

Mental Health Benefits - Medicare Advantage

Reviewing the plan's evidence of coverage documents is important to understand your mental health benefits under a Medicare Advantage plan. While coverage may vary, most Medicare Advantage plans adhere to the same 190-day lifetime limit for inpatient care in a psychiatric hospital.

Therapy Services - Limits

Medicare Part B covers therapy services such as physical therapy, speech-language pathology, and occupational therapy. As of 2019, there is no longer a limit on the coverage for therapy services in any given year. Medicare now covers outpatient treatment at 80% of the Medicare-approved amount. After meeting the Part B deductible of $198 in 2020, patients are responsible for a 20% co-pay when seeing a participating provider. If ongoing therapy is required for conditions such as stroke or heart disease, Medicare may continue to cover these services beyond the annual limits if the therapist justifies the need. Medicare automatically reviews cases when the total cost reaches $3,000 annually.

Co-Payments and Deductibles

The Part B deductible in 2020 was $198, typically adjusted slightly higher each year. Medicare covers 80% of the Medicare-approved cost for Part B services, and patients are responsible for the remaining 20%. However, if you receive care from a provider who does not accept the Medicare-approved cost as full payment, you may be charged more than 20%.

Limits on Out-of-Pocket Costs

Under traditional Medicare, Part B has no maximum cap on out-of-pocket expenses. However, if you have Medigap supplemental insurance, your Part B co-pays will be fully or partially covered based on your purchase policy.

Cost of Part D

Part D covers prescription drugs prescribed by a doctor and taken by the patient at home. To access this coverage, you can enroll in a standalone Part D drug plan if you have traditional Medicare for your medical benefits. Alternatively, you can choose a Medicare Advantage plan with medical and Part D drug coverage within its benefits package.

Chapter 3
Your Costs in Medicare

Topics:

- **Understanding Medicare Costs:** Learn about the expenses associated with Medicare, such as premiums, deductibles, and co-payments.
- **Higher Premiums Based on Income:** Discover how income levels can impact the premiums paid for Medicare coverage.
- **Factors Affecting Premium Differences:** Explore the factors that can cause premiums to vary among Medicare beneficiaries in different years.
- **Continued Medicare Tax Payments:** Gain insights into the obligation to pay Medicare taxes even after becoming a program beneficiary.

Understanding the Costs of Medicare

For individuals entering Medicare, one of the primary concerns is understanding how much it will cost and how much it will save them. The answer to this question largely depends on their previous insurance situation. If they had low-cost employer insurance, Medicare might appear expensive. However, if they had to pay high premiums for inadequate individual coverage or couldn't afford insurance, Medicare may be a relief.

It's important to note that Medicare is not free, and paying Medicare payroll taxes during employment does not guarantee free healthcare after turning 65. On average, Medicare covers only about half of beneficiaries' healthcare costs without additional insurance.

Premiums, Deductibles, and Co-payments

Medicare's coverage involves the medical care it provides, while the expenses that beneficiaries pay out of pocket come from premiums, deductibles, and co-payments. You likely understand these terms if you're already familiar with U.S.-style health insurance. However, if you're not, here's a brief explanation:

Premium: This is the monthly amount you pay for coverage or access to the Medicare program.

Deductible: This is the amount you must pay out of pocket before your coverage begins. It's similar to a down payment before receiving goods or services.

Co-payment: This is the fixed dollar amount you pay for each service you receive. In the past, you may have paid a single premium for all your healthcare needs, a yearly deductible, and co-pays for each service. However, Medicare is divided into four parts (A, B, D, and C), each with its costs and charges.

The following sections of the chapter will provide detailed information on the costs associated with Medicare Parts A, B, D, and C (Medicare Advantage plans). Additionally, Figure 3-1 will give you a quick overview of the costs for Parts A, B, and D. Note that these costs are for individuals enrolled in traditional Medicare with standalone Part D drug plans. Medicare Advantage plan costs may vary depending on the specific plan.

	Part A	**Part B**	**Part D**
Premiums	None if you or your spouse has earned 40 or more work credits by paying payroll taxes. $458 a month if you or your spouse has 30-39 credits. $252 a month if you or your spouse has 0-29 credits	For most people: $144.60 a month depending on circumstances. If you're liable for higher-income surcharges, you pay premiums of between $202.40 and $491.60 a month, depending on income level	Premiums vary among Part D plans, from about $15 to $230 a month, with most in the $35 to $55 a month range. If you're liable for higher-income premiums, you pay an additional surcharge of between $12.20 and $76.40 a month, depending on income level
Deductible	$1.408 for each hospital benefit period	Annual deductible: $198	Annual deductible: $0.00 to $435, depending on the p
Co-payments	Hospital stays: **Days 1-60:** No co-pays after deductible are met. **Days 61-90**: $352 a day in each benefit period. **Days 91-150:** $704 a day for each lifetime Reserve a day. <u>Skilled nursing facility</u>: Days 1-20: No co-pays. Days 21-100: $176 a day in each benefit period. After 100 days: You pay all costs.	None for most preventive services. 20 percent of the Medicare-approved cost for other services, unless you have other insurance that covers those costs.	Co-pays depend on what your plan charges for each drug and which phase of coverage you're in at any given point of the year.

FIGURE 3-1: At a glance, 2020 premiums, deductibles, and co-payments.

Costs Associated with Part A

Medicare Part A covers hospital and expert nursing facility care, hospice care, and home health services. However, there are certain expenses that you may need to pay out of pocket for these services.

The following sections will outline these potential costs, but it's important to note that they apply only to those enrolled in the traditional Medicare program. If you are in a Medicare Advantage health plan, such as an HMO or PPO, the costs may vary and will be discussed in a later section on "Medicare Advantage costs."

Premiums

Part A coverage does not require any premiums if you or your spouse have gained at least 40 credits (or quarters) through Medicare payroll taxes while working. However, if you need more credits through your or your spouse's work record, you can obtain Part A services by paying premiums. In 2020, the premium cost was $252 per month for individuals with 30 to 39 credits and $458 for those with less than 30 credits. These amounts are subject to annual adjustments.

Deductible

Unlike other parts of Medicare, Part A does not have an annual deductible. Instead, it applies a deductible to each hospital benefit period, which begins when you are admitted and ends when you have not been in the hospital for 60 consecutive days. Although this timeline may be confusing, it's important to know that the deductible for each hospital benefit period was $1,408 in 2020 and increases slightly each year. After you meet this deductible, Medicare covers the entire cost for up to 60 days.

Co-payments (hospital-skilled nursing facility)

If you stay in the hospital for over 60 days in a single benefit period, you will be liable for a daily co-pay from the 61st to the 90th day. 2020 this co-pay was $352 per day, increasing slightly each year. After 90 days, you can use some of your lifetime reserve days, subject to a substantial co-pay of $704 per day in 2020. You are limited to 60 reserve days for your entire life. Once you have used up these reserve days, you will be liable for paying your entire care cost.

Suppose you are transferred to a skilled nursing facility (SNF) after spending at least three days in the hospital. In that case, Medicare covers the entire cost for the first 20 days, and you are not responsible for any payment during this period. After that, you must pay a daily co-pay of $176 for up to 80 days. However, if you stay in the SNF for over 100 days in a single benefit period, you will be responsible for the entire cost. It is important to note that you cannot use your lifetime reserve days to extend coverage in an SNF.

Co-payments (Home Health Care - Hospice Care)

If you qualify for home health services, Medicare pays a home health agency for your care, and you pay nothing. However, if you need or want a service not covered under the agency contract, you must pay for it in whole or as a regular 20 percent Part B co-pay (see the later section on "Part B costs").

If you receive hospice services from a Medicare-approved agency, you pay almost nothing for this care, with two exceptions: If you need prescription drugs to control the symptoms, such as pain, of your terminal illness, you may have to pay up to $5 per prescription. If you need to enter a nursing home briefly so your caregiver can take a break, you are expected to contribute 5 percent of the cost.

Out-of-Pocket Limits

Medicare does not impose a yearly cap on your Part A expenses. However, supplemental insurance like a Medigap policy may cover the deductible and co-pays associated with Part A hospital services.

Costs Associated with Part B

Under Part B, Medicare covers expenses for doctors' services in their offices, hospitals, or at home. It also covers outpatient care, such as lab tests, screenings, and medical equipment and supplies. It's important to note that the following costs apply to traditional Medicare. If you're registered in a Medicare Advantage plan, you'll need to refer to the later section on "Medicare Advantage costs."

Premiums

To receive services under Part B, you must pay a monthly premium unless you are eligible for state assistance. The federal government announces the standard premium amount for the following year, typically in autumn. In 2020, the standard premium was $144.60 per month. However, this amount can vary based on income thresholds and Social Security cost-of-living adjustments. The annual Part B deductible for 2020 was $198, and it typically increases slightly each year, announced alongside the Part B premium.

Medicare normally covers 80 percent of the Medicare-approved cost of Part B services, while the beneficiary pays the remaining 20 percent. However, if a provider does not accept the Medicare-approved cost as full payment, the beneficiary may be charged more than 20 percent. Traditional Medicare has no upper limit on out-of-pocket expenses for Part B services. However, Medigap supplemental insurance may cover Part B co-pays fully or partially, depending on the specific policy purchased.

Costs Associated with Part D

Part D is a Medicare program that covers prescription drugs for outpatient use, prescribed by a doctor and usually taken at home. Suppose you have traditional Medicare for your medical benefits. In that case, you can get Part D coverage by signing up for a standalone Part D drug plan or enrolling in a Medicare Advantage plan that offers both medical and Part D drug coverage.

Premiums

Every standalone Part D plan requires a monthly premium, which can vary widely among plans. In 2020, premiums ranged from as low as $12.20 up to $76.40 per month, with the majority charging around $32. Most Medicare Advantage plans combine medical and drug services into a single premium; some plans have no premiums. It's important to note that both types of plans can alter their premiums each calendar year. The annual Part D deductible cannot exceed a certain amount each year, whether you're enrolled in a standalone or Medicare Advantage plan. In 2020, the maximum deductible was $435. However, many plans charge lower amounts or even waive the deductible.

Co-payments

Your Part D co-pays are determined by the amount your plan charges for each specific drug you take and the phase of coverage you are in during Part D's annual cycle. The co-pays can vary among different plans and may change each year. There is no flat cap on drug expenses in any year under Part D, but if your costs exceed a certain level, you may qualify for catastrophic coverage, where your drugs cost no more than 5% of the total price. Catastrophic coverage requires significant out-of-pocket spending.

Medicare Advantage Costs

Under Medicare Advantage, you can receive your Medicare benefits through a private health plan such as an HMO or PPO instead of traditional Medicare. If you enroll in a Medicare Advantage plan, you must accept its terms, conditions, and specific costs. Most plans require a monthly premium in addition to the one you pay for Part B services. The number of Medicare Advantage plan choices and average monthly premiums can vary yearly. In 2020, the average monthly premiums decreased by 14% to $23 from $26.87 in 2019. It's important to compare different plans to find the one that best suits your needs.

Deductible

While most Medicare Advantage plans do not have deductibles for medical services other than the standard Part B deductible, some plans may have them. The average deductible for Medicare Advantage plans in 2020 was $1,408. Further, plans that propose prescription drug coverage may have an annual deductible for Part D drugs, up to $435 in 2020, although some plans may charge less or none. Hospital stays typically do not have deductibles in most Medicare Advantage plans.

Co-payments

In several ways, co-pays in Medicare Advantage plans differ from those in traditional Medicare. Some plans charge a flat dollar co-pay for each medical service, whereas traditional Medicare charges a percentage of the cost. However, co-pays based on percentages are becoming more common in Medicare Advantage plans. Co-pays can vary significantly from plan to plan and can change from year to year. However, the amount charged for a specific service in January must remain the same for the rest of the year. PPOs and other plans may charge higher co-pays if you receive care outside their contracted networks. Unlike traditional Medicare, most Medicare Advantage plans do not charge a fixed deductible for hospital stays. Instead, they charge daily co-pays, which can vary greatly from plan to plan

Plans that offer vision, hearing, and dental care may charge co-pays for these services or offer them as optional packages that require an additional premium. Medicare Advantage plans cannot charge more than traditional Medicare for some services, such as chemotherapy for cancer, dialysis for kidney failure, and medical equipment.

Out-Of-Pocket Limits

In contrast to traditional Medicare, Medicare Advantage plans must set yearly limits on the expenses for the services covered by the plan that enrolled individuals pay annually. The limits can differ depending on the plan type and whether the cost is in-network or out-of-network. Contact the plan for further information.

Income-Related Premium Surcharge

Since its inception, Medicare has charged everyone the same premium for its services without means-testing. Even today, Medicare coverage is not denied based on an individual's wealth. However, individuals with incomes above a particular level have been required to pay higher premiums for Part B since 2007 because of the 2003 Medicare Modernization Act. Additionally, under the 2010 Affordable Care Act, these individuals must pay more for Part D.

This means that individuals who pay these higher premiums receive a smaller subsidy from the federal government for their healthcare.

The income they received two years before is considered to determine whether an individual needs to pay surcharges. For instance, whether an individual pays surcharges on their 2020 premiums is calculated based on their income in 2018, as reported on their tax returns filed in 2019.

The revised, altered gross income (MAGI) is the term the IRS uses to calculate the surcharge. The amount of income left after certain deductions excluded from the adjusted gross income (AGI), such as tax-exempt interest and student loan deductions, are added back in. Although it's a complicated calculation, the MAGI is often less than the full income.

Individuals whose income changes significantly in two years, such as those who have retired or lost their jobs, are not liable for the surcharge and can take action to avoid paying it.

Several factors can push some individuals above the surcharge threshold, even if their regular income is relatively modest, such as a one-year increase in income from the sale of property or cash in part or all of a tax-deferred asset like an individual retirement account (IRA) or selling stocks and shares.

Additionally, a one-year increase in income from a windfall, such as an inheritance, can result in surcharge liability. Such boosts to income in just one year can lead to a premium surcharge, but it won't be permanent. The following year, premiums will be based on regular income.

Your 2018 MAGI (Per 2019 Returns)	Your Part B Monthly Premium in 2020	Your Part D Monthly Premium in 2020
Single person: $87,000 or less Standard 2020 pre- Your regular Part D Married couple $144.60 plan premium filing jointly: $174,000 or less	Standard 2020 premium: $144.60	Your regular Part D plan premium
Single person: $87,000 to $109,000 Married couple filing jointly:	Standard 2020 premium: $202.40	Your Part D plan premium plus $12.20

$174,000 to $218,000 Single person: $109,000 to $136,000 Married couple filing jointly: $218,000 to $272,000	Standard 2020 premium: $289.20	Your Part D plan premium plus $31.50
Single person: $136,000 to $163,000 Married couple filing jointly: $272,000 to $326,000	Standard 2020 premium: $376.00	Your Part D plan premium plus $50.70
Single person: $163,000 to $500,000 Married couple filing jointly: $326,000 to	Standard 2020 premium: $462.70	Your Part D plan premium plus $70.00

$750,000		
Single person: $500,000 or above Married couple filing jointly: $750,000 or above	Standard 2020 premium: $491.60	Your Part D plan premium plus $76.40

TABLE 3-1 2020 Higher-Income Part B and Part D Premiums

Several factors can push some individuals above the surcharge threshold, even if their regular income is relatively modest, such as a one-year increase in revenue from the sale of property or cash in part or all of a tax-deferred asset like an individual retirement account (IRA) or selling stocks and shares. Additionally, a one-year increase in income from a windfall, such as an inheritance, can result in surcharge liability. Such boosts to income in just one year can lead to a premium surcharge, but it won't be permanent. The following year, premiums will be based on regular income.

Source: Centers for Medicare and Medicaid Services

Table 3-1 does not display an additional computation that pertains to married couples who file separate tax returns. In this scenario, each spouse must pay an additional fee based on their individual MAGI and falls into one of two categories: those earning between $87,000 and $413,000 and those earning $413,000 and above.

Because the surcharges are calculated as a percentage of the total expenses of Part B and Part D in the preceding year, the surcharges' precise dollar values alter slightly yearly. This is because the expenses may vary from year to year. However, the MAGI thresholds that determine the higher premium levels have remained unchanged up to 2019, and since 2020, they have been adjusted annually for inflation.

Surcharges Waived

A lot can happen in the two years that pass between the year in which your income is assessed and the year in which surcharges are applied. For example, in the former (I'll call it year A), you may be working and pulling in high earnings. In contrast, in the second scenario, where you're retired and have a considerably reduced income in year B, or in the event of being widowed or divorced or experiencing a stock market crash resulting in significant financial loss, you may wonder if the higher-income premium surcharges can be waived.

However, the following sections clarify the circumstances under which the Social Security Administration may grant waivers for these surcharges, as they are responsible for their assessment (not Medicare). Understanding life-changing events that qualify for waivers: The Social Security Administration recognizes situations where recent income changes may entitle you to avoid paying the higher-income premium surcharge.

These circumstances, which the administration calls "life-changing events," include:

- Marriage, divorce, annulment, or widowhood
- Retirement or job loss by you or your spouse
- Reduced work hours by you or your spouse
- Loss of income due to changes or termination of your former employer's pension plan
- Receiving a settlement due to your current or previous employer's closure, bankruptcy, or reorganization does not count toward a premium surcharge.
- Loss of income-generating assets (such as rented property, farmland, or livestock) resulting from an uncontrollable disaster or event.

Suppose you have experienced any of these circumstances resulting in decreased income and are currently paying the premium surcharge or have been informed that you will have to pay it soon. In that case, it is advisable to immediately contact the Social Security

Administration at 800-772-1213 or TTY 800-325-0778 and request a new initial determination.

Social Security will then evaluate whether you must pay the surcharge without needing a formal appeal. To obtain a new initial determination, you must furnish evidence of the life-changing event that triggered it, such as a death certificate or a letter from your previous employer confirming your job termination. Additionally, you must provide Social Security with a more recent tax return that verifies your decreased MAGI. If you still need to file a tax return for the current year, you must estimate your reduced earnings and provide a signed copy of the return to Social Security after filing it with the IRS.

To request a new initial determination and avoid paying higher-income premium surcharges, you should contact Social Security as soon as possible at 800-772-1213 or TTY 800-325-0778 if you have experienced a life-changing event resulting in reduced income. This can include marriage, divorce, retirement, loss of job, or receiving a settlement due to an employer's closure or bankruptcy. You must provide proper event documentation and evidence of reduced MAGI when requesting.

Social Security will process the request on the same day it is received if supported by proper documentation; otherwise, it may be delayed or denied. If Social Security determines that a life-changing event involves you, it will revise its records and waive or reduce the premium surcharges. This process may take some time, but any overpayments made will be refunded. If your proposal is declined, you can file an appeal by calling Social Security.

For example, Kate's retirement qualified as a life-changing event, allowing her to apply for a reassessment and reduce her premiums. Jose's sudden death counted as a life-changing event for his wife Maria, who was able to have her premiums reduced to the standard rate.

Other Situations Qualify for a Waiver

What if your income decreases due to other circumstances? For instance, what if you experienced a loss of investment income after a stock market crash? Even if it appears to be a life-changing event, Social Security does not consider it as such, and you cannot request a new determination. Your only option is to file an amended tax return with the IRS and present it to Social Security as proof of your reduced MAGI.

There is one more situation that is worth noting. Social Security may consider waiving the premium surcharge if your income is reduced due to fraud or criminal activity, such as falling victim to a Ponzi scheme. However, you must provide evidence of a crime or fraud and demonstrate that the perpetrator has been convicted.

If you can't qualify for a waiver based on a life-changing event but still can't afford to pay the premium surcharge due to loss of income, you may have to bear the higher premium until your next tax return reflects your reduced income. However, if paying the premiums causes severe financial hardship, Social Security may consider waiving the surcharge. You can contact Social Security and request a waiver if you're facing such a situation.

Paying Different Premiums

Occasionally, there are specific years when many Medicare beneficiaries pay one Part B premium while the remaining 30 percent pay a much higher amount. This is not related to the higher-income premium mentioned earlier but rather due to Social Security not providing a cost-of-living adjustment (COLA) or only a tiny one in some years. Under the law, individuals who receive Social Security benefits are protected from having their payments cut due to increased Part B premiums. Therefore, if there is no Social Security COLA each year and the Part B premium increases, these individuals are "held harmless," suggesting that the addition is waived, and they do not have to pay higher premiums than the previous year.

However, another long-established law requires Part B premiums to be set to cover about 25 percent of expected costs in the program for the upcoming year. When costs increase, premiums rise. Who pays if the people who are held harmless cannot contribute to the increase? Everyone else on Medicare, including those who do not receive Social Security or Railroad Retirement benefits, those who are new to Medicare, and those who pay higher income-related premiums. Lower-income beneficiaries who receive Medicaid or whose Part B premiums are paid by their state are unaffected as their state pays the increased premium, not the beneficiary.

The Medicare Hold Harmless provision is in place to ensure that individuals who receive Social Security do not see significant reductions in their monthly payments when Medicare Part B premiums outpace the cost-of-living adjustment (COLA) each year. In some years, those held harmless pay less than the standard premium while everyone else pays the total amount. For example, in 2016 and 2017, those held harmless paid $104.90 and a few dollars above that amount, respectively, while the standard premium was $121.80 and a record $134. In 2020, a 1.6 percent COLA adjustment was less than the 2.8 percent adjustment in 2019. Still, it increased the average beneficiary's total benefit by about $24 a month, which should cover the roughly $9 increase in Part B premiums.

The Consumer Price Index (CPI) calculates the Social Security COLA, indicating overall inflation in consumer prices. In certain years, such as 2010, 2011, and 2016, the CPI indicated no inflation or deflation, primarily due to decreased oil prices. Although the CPI for 2020 is 1.3 percent, much lower than the peak of 2.13 percent in 2017, it does not account for healthcare expenses, which constitute a significant portion of the everyday costs for Americans, especially those eligible for Medicare.

Paying Medicare Taxes While Receiving Medicare Benefits:

I have been asked this question frequently: "As someone over 65 still working and enrolled in Medicare, should my employer continue to deduct Medicare payroll taxes from my earnings?" Indeed, if you are under 65 and still working, your employer must legally withhold Social Security and Medicare taxes from your wages. If your employer has stopped doing so, you should discuss this matter with your employer or call the Social Security Administration to determine the appropriate course of action.

It is essential to continue paying Medicare and Social Security taxes even if your employer has stopped deducting them. Failure to do so could put your future benefits at risk. Unfortunately, this situation is not uncommon, and some employers wrongly believe they can classify employees as independent contractors to avoid paying these taxes. The IRS warns that employee misclassification can lead to penalties for the business. However, this misclassification can significantly impact your earnings. As an employee, your employer must legally pay half of your Medicare and Social Security payroll taxes. You are responsible for paying the full amount if you are an independent contractor.

Chapter 4
Reducing Your Out-of-Pocket Expenses

Topics:

- Medigap supplemental insurance: Pay extra through Medigap premiums to lower costs in deductibles and co-pays
- Medicare Advantage: Join a Medicare Advantage plan to reduce costs
- State and federal assistance: Qualify for assistance based on a limited income to help pay for Medicare costs
- Extra Help program: Federal program providing Part D prescription drug coverage at a lower cost for eligible individuals
- Detailed exploration of Medigap, state and federal assistance programs, and other cost-cutting strategies
- Practical tips to navigate these options and reduce out-of-pocket costs associated with Medicare.

Exploring Medigap Insurance Options

Medigap, also known as Medicare supplemental insurance, is a private insurance choice that can help lower expenses in the traditional Medicare program. If you lack additional coverage like retirement benefits and can afford extra premiums, Medigap is worth considering. It covers a significant portion of co-pays and deductibles, with additional coverage based on the chosen policy.

Key Facts about Medigap

Medicare Part A and Part B enrollment is required for Medigap eligibility and cannot be used with Medicare Advantage plans. Besides the Part B premium, monthly premiums for Medigap coverage must be paid. Medigap policies generally do not cover prescription drug costs unless it is an older policy from before 2006.

If you are 65 or older, federal law provides consumer protections during specific enrollment periods, protecting against coverage refusal or higher premiums based on health conditions.

Individuals under 65 are not eligible for these federal protections, although some states offer similar rights.

Understanding Medigap Policies

Ten designated Medigap policies are marked as letters A, B, C, D, F, G, K, L, M, and N. (Letters E, H, I, and J are not used for newer policies.) These policies offer standardized benefits determined by federal law. Policies with the same letter provide identical benefits, but premiums may vary among insurance companies. Hence, comparing policies from different insurers is advisable.

Figure 4-1 provides an overview of the benefits covered by each Medigap policy and the extent of coverage. The percentages indicate the portion of a benefit's cost that the policy pays, with the individual responsible for the remainder. However, it is crucial to review policy details as there may be limitations or additional costs not depicted in the chart. For instance, the emergency care abroad benefit has undisclosed limits. Six policies covering this benefit have a $250 deductible, a 20% co-pay, and a $ 50,000 lifetime limit.

Furthermore, the Part B excess charges benefit is exclusive to policies F and G, addressing expenses when providers charge more than the Medicare-approved cost. This is known as balance billing. It should be noted that new Medicare beneficiaries no longer have access to supplemental Plan F policies.

Covered Benefits	*A*	*B*	*C*	*D*	*F*	*G*	*K*	*L*	*M*	*N*
Part A hospital co-pays plus 365 extra days	**Yes**	**Yes**	**Yes**	**Yes**	**Yes**	**Yes**	**Yes**	**Yes**	**Yes**	**Yes**
Part A hospital deductible	*No*	**Yes**	**Yes**	**Yes**	**Yes**	**Yes**	*50%*	*75%*	*50%*	**Yes**
Part B co-pays	**Yes**	**Yes**	**Yes**	**Yes**	**Yes**	**Yes**	*50%*	*75%*	**Yes**	**Yes**
Part B deductible	*No*	*No*	**Yes**	*No*	**Yes**	*No*	*No*	*No*	*No*	*No*
Part B excess charges	*No*	*No*	*No*	*No*	**Yes**	**Yes**	*No*	*No*	*No*	*No*
Skilled nursing facility co-pays	*No*	*No*	**Yes**	**Yes**	**Yes**	**Yes**	*50%*	*75%*	**Yes**	**Yes**
Hospice care co-pays	**Yes**	**Yes**	**Yes**	**Yes**	**Yes**	**Yes**	*50%*	*75%*	**Yes**	**Yes**
First 3 pints of blood	**Yes**	**Yes**	**Yes**	**Yes**	**Yes**	**Yes**	*50%*	*75%*	**Yes**	**Yes**
Emergency care abroad (to plan limits)	*No*	*No*	**Yes**	**Yes**	**Yes**	**Yes**	*No*	*No*	**Yes**	**Yes**

FIGURE 4-1: Benefits covered in Medigap policies.

Policy N covers most of the 20% co-pays under Part B, but some exceptions require small co-pays. For certain office visits, the co-pay can be up to $20; for emergency room visits without hospital admission, it can be up to $50.

Policies K and L, on the other hand, cover only half or three-fourths of the costs for most services. However, if your out-of-pocket expenses exceed certain annual limits, they will cover 100% of your costs for the rest of the year. Some states offer an alternative high-deductible version of policy F, with lower premiums but a substantial annual deductible. In 2020, the deductible was $2,340 before the policy provided coverage. This deductible can vary from year to year. The standard F policy does not have a deductible.

Certain policies have a "SELECT" version with lower premiums but limited coverage to network providers, except for emergencies.

Previously, policies C and F covered the annual Part B deductible of $198 in 2020. However, this benefit was discontinued for policies sold from 2020 onwards. When purchasing Medigap, it's important to compare the details of each policy to make an informed decision.

Living in Massachusetts, Minnesota, or Wisconsin

These states had established standardized Medigap policies before the federal law. While the benefits are similar to national policies, there are some differences. For example, Wisconsin offers additional mental health coverage and home health visits, while Minnesota provides a benefit for physical therapy. Residents in these states have fewer policy options than other parts of the country. To find out available policies and specific benefits, residents can use the Medigap plan finder program on Medicare's website by entering their zip code.

Having a Medigap Policy, That's No Longer Sold

Over time, Medigap insurance has changed to enhance consumer protection. Some policies, such as E, H, I, and J, have been paused and are no longer available to new customers. However, existing policyholders can continue using these policies and maintain the original benefits, although premiums may increase. The rise in premiums is due to a decreasing number of policyholders with the same policy, resulting in higher costs for the insurance company.

Policies H, I, and J used to include coverage for prescription drugs when Medicare didn't provide it. However, since Medicare prescription drug coverage (Part D) was introduced in 2006, these policies were no longer sold. Policyholders had the option to remove the drug coverage or switch to a Medigap policy without drug coverage while enrolling in Part D. It's important to note that the drug coverage offered by these policies is not considered as good as Part D coverage, and switching to Part D later may result in permanent late penalties.

Choosing and Buying a Medigap Policy

After reviewing the available Medigap options, selecting a policy and insurance company that meet your needs is crucial. This chapter provides insights into the factors to consider when choosing a Medigap policy, the appropriate time to purchase one (age 65 or older with federal protections), and the importance of timing in terms of cost. Federal protections do not apply to individuals under 65, but some states may offer similar or alternative protections.

Qualifying for State Assistance

If you're facing difficulties affording the basic costs of Medicare, including Medigap options, there may be assistance available through your state. It's essential to explore all options for maintaining coverage, even if you're considering discontinuing premium payments. Many people who qualify for state programs must know their existence and how to apply. This section describes various types of assistance for individuals in financial need, such as Medicaid, Medicaid medical spend-down programs, Medicare Savings Programs (MSPs), Programs of All-Inclusive Care for the Elderly (PACE), and State Pharmacy Assistance Programs (SPAPs) to help cover prescription drug costs.

Medicaid

Medicaid is a government-funded program that delivers medical coverage to individuals with limited income, including seniors and people with disabilities. Currently, there are approximately 72 million enrollees in Medicaid, with more than one in five also enrolled in Medicare, known as dual eligibles. If you qualify for full Medicaid benefits, you can expect to pay little or nothing for medical expenses, as Medicaid covers your out-of-pocket costs in Medicare. Medicaid offers coverage for services not covered by Medicare, such as extended stays in skilled nursing facilities, hearing aids, eyeglasses, and long-term care in a nursing home.

Full Medicaid benefits automatically make you eligible for free or low-cost prescription drug scope through the Part D Extra Help program.

Each state administers Medicaid in collaboration with the federal government, and eligibility requirements may vary. Typically, eligibility is based on factors like monthly income, savings, residency, and citizenship or legal residency. The assessment of eligibility considers joint income for married individuals living with their spouse but individual income for those living in someone else's home unless claimed as a dependent on their tax returns.

Due to administrative barriers, navigating the eligibility process and finding Medicaid-accepting doctors can be challenging. Medicaid beneficiaries may experience loss of coverage in certain circumstances, and administrative barriers caused a quarter of Medicaid beneficiaries to become uninsured in 2019. If you are eligible for both Medicaid and Medicare, considering Special Needs Plans (SNPs) offered by Medicare Advantage plans may be beneficial. These plans are designed specifically for dual eligibles and coordinate services between Medicare and Medicaid for optimized benefits.

Medicaid Medical Spend-Down Programs

Certain states offer medical spend-down or medically needy programs that allow individuals with incomes exceeding the state's Medicaid limit to qualify once their out-of-pocket medical costs reach a specific threshold within a calendar year. Eligibility rules for these programs vary by state, and benefits are typically granted for a limited period, such as six months. After that period, individuals may need to restart the application process since their personal medical expenses decrease and no longer meet the eligibility criteria. However, if you have Medicaid through one of these programs, most of your out-of-pocket Medicare costs are covered, at least for specific periods.

You automatically qualify for full Extra Help, which provides low-cost Medicare drug coverage. Even if your Medicaid coverage ends earlier, once enrolled in the Extra Help program, you will continue to receive its benefits until at least the end of the calendar year. To determine if your state offers a medical spend-down program, contact your local Medicaid office or refer to Appendix A for your State Health Insurance Assistance Program (SHIP) contact information.

Medicare Savings Programs

Medicare Savings Programs (MSPs) provide assistance to individuals with income and savings below specific limits, which vary by state. These limits are generally higher than those for Medicaid qualification, and in some states, savings are not considered. It is recommended to apply for the MSP if you meet the criteria. MSPs are available in four types: Qualified Medicare Beneficiary (QMB), Specified Low Income Medicare Beneficiary (SLMB), Qualifying Individual (QI), and Qualified Disabled and Working Individuals (QDWI).

Each type has its own income limit and offers different coverage options, including Part B premium coverage and coverage for other Medicare costs such as deductibles and co-pays. Qualifying for an MSP, even if it only covers your Part B premium, automatically makes you eligible for full Extra Help under the Part D prescription drug program, resulting in significantly reduced medication costs. Another advantage of MSP eligibility is that if you have incurred a late penalty due to delayed enrollment in Part B, the state will pay your Part B premium, and the penalty will be waived.

State Pharmacy Assistance Programs (SPAPs) or Pharmaceutical Assistance Programs are available in twenty-four states and the U.S. Virgin Islands. These programs aim to help individuals with limited incomes cover the costs of prescription drugs when their income exceeds the eligibility threshold for Medicaid. Some SPAPs have higher income limits than those set by Medicare Part D's Extra Help program. Additionally, certain SPAPs do not consider your savings and resources, which may not affect your eligibility.

The benefits provided by SPAPs vary among different programs. Some programs offer a comprehensive range of services that complement the Extra Help program, assisting Part D enrollees who don't qualify for Extra Help. Other programs focus on helping patients with specific medical conditions, such as cancer, or provide discount cards for pharmacy use.

When you regularly need many medications or face high costs for expensive drugs, prescription expenses can become a significant financial burden. While the Part D prescription drug program provides some assistance, expenses such as premiums, deductibles, co-pays, and the coverage gap (also known as the "doughnut hole") can accumulate and become unaffordable. This is where Extra Help comes in.

Extra Help is a unique program within Part D that offers low-cost drug coverage and eliminates the coverage gap. It specifically targets individuals with incomes and savings below a certain threshold. Extra Help has provided significant financial relief to millions of Medicare beneficiaries, allowing them to save hundreds and thousands of dollars annually on prescription drug expenses. It has also enabled individuals without prior drug coverage to access the medications they need for the first time.

To qualify for Extra Help, you may need to apply depending on your circumstances. Full Extra Help is automatically granted if you have full Medicaid coverage, Supplemental Security Income (SSI), your state pays your Medicare premiums, or qualify for a Medicaid medical spend-down program. You'll need to apply for Extra Help if you still need to meet these criteria.

Extra Help has five eligibility levels, with the first three based solely on income. Levels four and five require filling out an application that asks for details about your income and assets, notably savings. Each level has its eligibility requirements and associated costs. If you believe your income falls just below the specified limits, applying regardless is recommended. Income limits can be higher in certain situations, such as having earnings from work that aren't considered, residing in Alaska or Hawaii, or having dependent relatives living with you.

To apply for Extra Help, complete a form and submit it to the Social Security Administration. The form can be obtained online through the Social Security website, by phone from Social Security, in person at a local Social Security or State Health Insurance Assistance Program (SHIP) office, or through automatic mailing from Social Security.

Choose the most convenient method to obtain the Extra Help application form.

What Qualifies as Income? When completing the application form, ensure that you provide all relevant information related to the following:

- Earnings from self-employment or pre-tax wages

- Social Security or railroad retirement benefits before deductions
- Veterans' benefits
- Pensions and annuities
- Workers' compensation
- Alimony
- Net income from rental property

However, you can exclude the following information:

- Cash or credit obtained through a loan or reverse mortgage
- Federal income tax refunds and earned income tax credit payments
- Victims' compensation
- Education grants and scholarships
- Assistance received from food stamps, a housing agency, an energy assistance program, or a public relocation program
- Support received from someone contributing to your food, mortgage, rent, heating fuel, gas, electricity, water, and property taxes
- Assistance provided for medical treatment and drugs
- Disaster assistance

Include the necessary details for the listed items and omit any information that does not apply to your situation when filling out the form.

What Qualifies as Assets? Assets, also known as resources, refer to the value of certain possessions you own, primarily savings. When reporting your assets, include any of the following items that you possess:

- Bank accounts, including checking, savings, and certificates of deposit
- Proceeds from a loan if saved beyond the month received
- Cash kept at home or in another location
- Individual retirement accounts (IRAs) and 401(K)s
- Stocks, bonds, and mutual funds
- Real estate properties (excluding your primary home)

However, you can exclude the following items from your list of assets:

- Your primary home and the land it is situated on
- Your vehicle(s)
- Personal possessions such as jewelry and furnishings
- Property essential for self-support, such as land used for growing your own food

- Burial plots
- Life insurance policies

When completing the application, include the relevant assets while excluding those that do not apply to your situation.

Regarding Social Security's Extra Help program, there are no restrictions on spending down or gifting a portion of your savings to bring them below the asset limit. Only the assets you possess at the time of your application are considered. However, keep in mind that giving away or spending down assets may affect your eligibility for other assistance programs, especially Medicaid, as it has specific guidelines in this regard. This is particularly important if you anticipate needing such programs within a few years.

What Constitutes "Single" and "Married" for Income Purposes? The income thresholds set by Social Security for Extra Help apply to single individuals and married couples living together, regardless of gender. If you are married and residing together, you can apply together using a single form. However, if only one of you is applying, you still need to provide information about your spouse's income and assets. You are considered single if you are living apart, have a spouse permanently living in a long-term care facility, or have a domestic partner. However, if you are in a common-law marriage, it is advisable to consult with Social Security as the recognition of your marital status may depend on the laws of your state.

What if I'm Supporting Other Family Members? Make sure to indicate the number of family members living with you who rely on you or your spouse for at least 50% of their support, including relatives related to you by blood, marriage, or adoption. The more people you support, the higher the income limits, increasing your likelihood of meeting the requirements for Extra Help.

Who Can Assist Me with the Application? If you find it challenging to complete the Extra Help application on your own due to circumstances such as illness or the recent loss of a spouse, you have several options available:

- **Seek assistance from someone you know:** A family member, friend, legal representative, social worker, or anyone you trust can help you complete the application or even apply on your behalf.
- **Obtain free, expert personal help:** Counselors at your State Health Insurance Assistance Program (SHIP) are trained to assist in navigating Part D options and applying for Extra Help. Refer to Appendix A for contact information for your SHIP.
- **Contact Social Security:** If you need help with specific questions, try calling Social Security at 800-772-1213 (TTY 800-325-0778). Or, visit your local Social Security office.
- **Engage community groups:** If you belong to a religious institution, senior center, or other community organization, they may provide assistance in completing the

application. For non-English speakers, organizations or groups catering to individuals of your nationality can be especially helpful. See Appendix A for non-English sources of assistance.

How Do I Complete the Application Process?

After completing and signing the form, you declare that the information provided is true and accurate to the best of your knowledge. If you are married and living together, your spouse also needs to sign it, even if they are not applying for Extra Help. If someone else signs on your behalf, they must fill out the section of the form that asks for their name, address, and their relationship to you. You can submit the form by mail using the pre-addressed envelope, apply online through Social Security, or apply on the BenefitsCheckUp website.

Once you have submitted your application, Social Security will send you a notice acknowledging receipt and confirming that they are processing it. If you do not receive this notice within a couple of weeks, contact Social Security to check the status of your application.

Social Security may contact you by phone or mail if they have additional questions or if your application is incomplete or inaccurate. If your application is likely to be denied, you may receive a pre-decisional notice outlining the reasons. This notice gives you the opportunity to correct any incorrect or incomplete information within ten days of the notice date by visiting or contacting your local Social Security office.

Social Security will determine your eligibility for Extra Help, and you should receive a response within 60 days of submitting your application. You'll receive either a Notice of Award or a Notice of Denial, depending on whether you qualify for full or partial Extra Help or are not eligible at all. If you disagree with the decision, the Notice of Denial will provide instructions on how to appeal.

What if Social Security Denies My Application?

If you disagree with Social Security's decision, you have the right to appeal. You must submit an appeal within 60 days of receiving the decision, and you have two options:

- **Request a telephone hearing:** Call your local Social Security office or the national number (800-772-1213 or TTY 800-325-0778) and ask for an appeal request form. Fill out the form and mail it in. Once your request is processed, you'll receive a letter with the date of your hearing and the number to call. You can also request a conference call if you want someone to assist you during the hearing. The letter will provide instructions on submitting additional documents supporting your case.
- **Ask for a case review:** A Social Security agent must review your application and any additional information you submit, but you will not be able to present your case in person. After the review, you'll receive a letter with the decision. If you win, you will receive Extra Help retroactive to the month in which you initially applied. If you lose

but still disagree with the decision, you can file a further appeal in a federal court within 60 days of receiving the letter.

If you are denied Extra Help on your current application, do not be discouraged from reapplying, especially if your income or assets were only slightly over the limits. Keep in mind that the limits increase slightly each year, and even a small decrease in your financial situation may make you eligible for Extra Help through a new application.

If I am eligible, how long will I receive Extra Help?

Typically, if you qualify for Extra Help, you will continue to receive it until the end of the current year, even if your financial situation changes during that year. However, whether you will continue to receive Extra Help from January 1 of the following year depends on whether your financial situation has improved.

If any of the following circumstances occur, you may lose Extra Help or receive a reduced benefit next year:

- If your income exceeds the limits for Extra Help.
- If the value of your savings and other countable assets exceeds the asset limits for Extra Help.
- If you no longer qualify for programs that automatically make you eligible for Extra Help, such as Medicaid or SSI, including your premiums paid by your state, or living in a Medicaid spend-down program.

If any of the following marital events occur during the year, you must report them immediately to have your Extra Help eligibility reviewed:

- If your spouse dies.
- If you and your partner separate, divorce, or have your marriage annulled.
- If you and your spouse reconcile after living apart.
- If you get married.

If any of these events happen to you, contact Social Security (800-772-1213 or TTY 800-325-0778) to report it and complete a redetermination form over the phone, in person at your local Social Security office, or via mail. If you complete the form within 90 days of filing the report, Social Security will determine whether to increase or reduce your Extra Help, terminate it, or leave it unchanged. Any changes will occur the following month after you've filed the report. However, complete the required form within 90 days to ensure your Extra Help benefit is not terminated.

How can I find out if my Extra Help will continue?

What happens next year and how you can find out depends on how you initially qualified for Extra Help, as explained below:

If you are automatically qualified for Extra Help: If your situation remains unchanged, there is nothing you need to do, and you will continue to receive the benefit. However, if you are no longer enrolled in Medicaid or SSI or your state is no longer paying your premiums, Medicare will send you a notice on gray paper informing you that you no longer qualify automatically for Extra Help but can still apply for it.

If you qualified for Extra Help through a Medicaid medical spend-down program: If your medical expenses continue to be high enough to remain enrolled in Medicaid at the end of the year, you will continue to receive Extra Help next year. If your medical expenses no longer qualify you for Medicaid, you will likely receive a letter informing you that your Extra Help benefit will end on January 1. Suppose your name is still in the system in July when Medicare compiles its list of automatically eligible individuals for Extra Help next year. In that case, you will receive benefits for the entire year.

If you applied for Extra Help: In August or September, you may receive a letter from Social Security asking whether your financial situation has changed. You must fill out the form and return it within 30 days if it has. If you return the form, your Extra Help will continue on December 31. Social Security will review your information and inform you if you still qualify for Extra Help next year and, if so, whether there will be any changes to your benefits.

For example, if your income has decreased, you may have lower co-pays next year. Conversely, if your income has increased beyond a certain level, you may only receive partial Extra Help instead of full Extra Help. Any changes to your benefits will take effect from January 1.

Choosing a drug plan with Extra Help: If you have Extra Help, it's important to select a Medicare prescription drug plan (Part D) that works well with your Extra Help benefits.

Here are some things to consider when selecting a drug plan:

Review your current coverage: Look at your current prescription drug plan and assess how well it meets your needs. Consider the medications you take regularly, the costs associated with your current plan, and any restrictions or limitations that may be in place.

Compare Part D plans: Use the Medicare Plan Finder tool on the official Medicare website (medicare.gov) to compare options in your area. Enter your zip code, medications, and dosage information for personalized results. The tool will show you a list of plans, their costs, and the pharmacies in their networks.

Look for plans with low premiums and deductibles: Since you have Extra Help, you should focus on finding plans with low premiums and deductibles. Extra Help can help cover the costs, but minimizing your out-of-pocket expenses is still beneficial.

Consider the formulary: Each Part D plan has a method: a list of covered medications. Make sure the plan you choose includes the specific medications you need. You can check each plan's formulary to ensure your medications are covered and determine any restrictions or prior authorization requirements.

Review cost-sharing and co-pays: Look into the cost-sharing structure of each plan, including co-pays or coinsurance for the medications you take. With Extra Help, you may qualify for reduced or even $0 co-pays for generic and brand-name drugs. Find a plan that offers affordable cost-sharing options for the medications you rely on.

Consider the pharmacy network: Check if your preferred pharmacy is included in the plan's network. Some plans have preferred pharmacies where you can get your medications at lower costs. If you have a specific pharmacy you prefer or need access to specialty pharmacies, ensure that they are within the plan's network.

Assess customer satisfaction and ratings: Look for plans with high ratings and positive customer reviews. Medicare provides ratings for Part D plans based on member satisfaction, customer service, and medication adherence. Consider choosing a plan with a good reputation and positive feedback.

Seek assistance if needed: If you find the process overwhelming or need help understanding the alternatives, speak with your local State Health Insurance Assistance Program (SHIP) for personalized assistance. They can guide you through the plan selection process and help you make an informed decision.

Remember to enroll in your chosen Part D plan during the annual Medicare Open Enrollment Period, typically from October 15 to December 7 each year. You can switch to a new Part D plan or change your existing one during this period. By carefully comparing Part D plans and considering your specific needs, you can find a plan that complements your Extra Help benefits and provides the necessary prescription drug coverage.

Switching to Less Expensive Medications: Consider transitioning to less expensive drugs that are equally effective for your medical conditions. Brand-name drugs, particularly the newest ones favored by doctors, tend to be the costliest. However, alternative versions are often available, such as generics or older brand-name drugs, that are equally effective but more affordable. While these alternatives may require slight adjustments, like taking multiple pills instead of one, they serve the same medical purpose. Consult your doctor about the viability of using a generic or older drug that is just as effective for your condition as the current brand-name medication.

Switching to a Lower-Cost Part D Drug Plan: Research shows that selecting an alternative Part D drug plan can lead to significant cost savings. Co-payments for the same medication can vary greatly among different plans, making it crucial to compare available plans each year based on your specific drug needs. By making informed decisions, you can reduce your expenses.

Using Mail Order or Preferred Pharmacies

Some Part D plans offer mail-order services that allow you to obtain a 90-day supply of medications at lower co-pays. However, verifying if this option is cost-effective for your specific drugs is important, as it may only sometimes result in savings. Utilizing a "preferred" pharmacy within your plan's network can reduce co-payment amounts. Check with your plan to see if they offer this benefit and obtain a list of preferred pharmacies in your area.

Finding Free or Low-Cost Prescription Drugs

There are possibilities worth exploring in situations where certain medications are still unaffordable, even with Part D coverage. Some drug manufacturers offer patient assistance programs that provide free or discounted supplies of their brand-name products under specific circumstances. Additionally, certified charities and patient organizations that assist individuals with specific medical conditions can provide support. It's important to exercise caution when considering purchasing drugs from abroad through mail orders due to the presence of scams. Other options include requesting free samples from your doctor or exploring pharmacy discounts, which can significantly reduce prices for selected drugs.

Part 2 - The How's and When's of Medicare

This section provides information on Medicare eligibility requirements and guidance on when to enroll based on individual circumstances. Understanding the enrollment rules is crucial to avoid permanent late penalties and coverage delays. It also covers practical aspects of the enrollment process, such as automatic enrollment, applying for Medicare, considerations for United States or abroad residents, and the commencement of coverage. The section also addresses how Medicare aligns with other health insurance plans, including coverage from employers, federal programs, veterans' programs, and various insurance types.

Eligibility for Medicare

To be eligible for Medicare, you must generally meet one of the following criteria:

Age-Based Eligibility: You qualify for Medicare if you are 65 years old or older and either a U.S. citizen or a permanent legal citizen who has lived in the United States for at least five consecutive years.

Disability-Based Eligibility: You may be eligible for Medicare if you are under 65 years old and have obtained Social Security Disability Insurance (SSDI) or Railroad Retirement Board disability benefits for a certain period (usually 24 months).

End-Stage Renal Disease (ESRD) or Amyotrophic Lateral Sclerosis (ALS): If you have ESRD (permanent kidney failure requiring dialysis or a kidney transplant) or ALS (also known as Lou Gehrig's disease), you are eligible for Medicare, regardless of your age.

Timing of Medicare Enrollment: The timing of your Medicare enrollment depends on your circumstances. Understanding the enrollment periods and deadlines is essential to ensure seamless coverage. Let's explore the different enrollment periods:

Initial Enrollment Period (IEP): If you become eligible for Medicare based on age, your IEP begins three months before your 65th birthday month. It ends three months after. Enrolling during this period is generally recommended to avoid any late enrollment penalties.

Special Enrollment Period (SEP): Certain situations may qualify you for a SEP, allowing you to enroll in or change your Medicare coverage outside the regular enrollment periods. Some common examples include losing employer-sponsored health coverage, moving out of your plan's service area, or qualifying for extra Help with Medicare prescription drug costs.

General Enrollment Period (GEP): If you missed your IEP and didn't qualify for a SEP, you can enroll in Medicare during the GEP, which runs from January 1 to March 31 each year. However, remember that late enrollment penalties may apply if you don't have creditable coverage (other prescription drug coverage considered at least as good as Medicare's) during the coverage gap.

Annual Enrollment Period (AEP): The AEP, also known as the Open Enrollment Period, happens from October 15 to December 7 each year. During this period, you can change your Medicare coverage by switching between Original Medicare and Medicare Advantage or changing your Part D prescription drug plan.

Enrollment Process: The enrollment process for Medicare depends on various factors, including whether you will be automatically enrolled or need to apply, your residency status, the availability of options to delay enrollment without penalties, and the timing of your coverage. Here are some key points to consider:

Automatic Enrollment: If you're already receiving Social Security or Railroad Retirement Board benefits, you will generally be automatically enrolled in Medicare Parts A and B when eligible. You will receive your Medicare card in the mail about three months before your 65th birthday or your 25th month of disability benefits.

Applying for Medicare: If you're not automatically enrolled, you must apply for Medicare through the Social Security Administration. You can apply online, by phone, or visiting your local Social Security office.

Residency and Enrollment: If you live in the United States, you can generally enroll in Medicare. However, the enrollment rules may vary if you reside outside the U.S. It's advisable to contact the Social Security Administration or visit their website for detailed information.

Delaying Enrollment: If you have other credible health coverage, such as through an employer or union, you may be able to delay enrolling in Medicare without incurring late penalties. It's important to evaluate your options carefully and assess whether delaying enrollment is right for you.

Coverage Start Date: Your coverage start date will depend on when you enroll. If you enroll during your IEP, your coverage typically begins on the first day of your birthday month or the month after you enroll. If you register during the GEP, your coverage will start on July 1 of the year you enrolled. Be aware that exceptions and variations may vary depending on your situation.

Medicare and Other Health Insurance: Medicare works in coordination with other health insurance plans you may have, such as coverage from your current or former employer, the Federal Employees Health Benefits Program, the Veterans Affairs health program, the military's TRICARE programs, the Indian Health Service, the federal Black Lung Program, the Workers' Compensation program, as well as no-fault and liability insurance. Understanding how Medicare aligns with these plans will help make informed decisions about your healthcare coverage.

Please note that the information provided here is a general overview, and it's essential to consult official Medicare resources, such as the official Medicare website, or contact the Social Security Administration for specific details and guidance based on your unique circumstances.

Chapter 5
Qualifying for Medicare

Topics

- Gaining a comprehensive understanding of the requirements for Medicare eligibility at the age of 65.
- Exploring the process of becoming eligible for Medicare before the age of 65 due to a disability.
- Analyzing alternative healthcare options for individuals who are not yet eligible for Medicare.

Qualifying for Medicare and being eligible for Medicare essentially indicate the same thing: you have fulfilled the necessary legal criteria to receive Medicare benefits. Rest assured, there is no examination or formal ceremony required to qualify for Medicare. There is no need to appear before a judge or go through any elaborate process. However, you must meet specific conditions outlined by the law.

In broad terms, there are two main conditions you must satisfy:

You have reached the age of 65 (or will do so very soon) or are older than 65.

You are under 65 but have an officially recognized disability that meets the requirements for Medicare coverage.

Within these two categories, various other conditions exist that may or may not apply to your specific situation. In this chapter, I will provide a detailed explanation of all these conditions. Additionally, I will outline the options available for healthcare if you do not immediately qualify for Medicare at the age of 65, if you are a few years away from turning 65, or if you find yourself in the two-year waiting period that individuals under 65 and disabled typically face before receiving Medicare coverage.

Hitting the Milestone of Age 65

Reaching the age of 65 is a significant milestone that can feel more like a monumental leap than a mere distance traveled. (Where did all the time go, indeed?) Regardless of how it may be perceived by the baby boomer generation, whose mantra once cautioned against trusting anyone over 30, turning 65 bestows a valuable gift in the form of assured healthcare coverage through Medicare.

However, it's important to note that simply reaching the age of 65 does not automatically qualify you for Medicare. Additional conditions must be met, depending on your specific circumstances, which I will elaborate on in the following sections. Furthermore, I will address common misconceptions surrounding Medicare eligibility, providing clarity on the matter.

Debunking some qualification myths

I want to clarify the true meaning of "qualifying for Medicare" to avoid any misunderstandings. Many individuals believe that if they haven't contributed enough through payroll taxes during their working years, they are not eligible for any Medicare benefits. However, this belief is incorrect. Payroll taxes primarily cover the premiums for Part A, allowing individuals to receive Part A services without additional monthly premiums. However, even if you are not entitled to premium-free Part A, you can still access Part B and Part D services by paying the required premiums like everyone else.

Furthermore, even if you have not worked enough to qualify for premium-free Part A, there may still be options available to you. For instance, you might qualify based on the work record of your current, divorced, or deceased spouse. Alternatively, you may have the choice to receive Part A benefits by paying monthly premiums for them.

I would also like to clarify a few other points that often lead to confusion:

- The law does not mandate that you must enroll in Medicare Part B (which requires monthly premiums) at the age of 65 or any other age. The decision to enroll is entirely up to you. However, it's important to note that if you later change your mind after the enrollment deadline has passed, you may face costly consequences in the form of late penalties.
- You have the option to enroll in Medicare at the age of 65 or later, even if you have not yet started receiving Social Security or railroad retirement benefits.
- You can choose to delay enrolling in Part B beyond the age of 65 without incurring late penalties if you have health insurance coverage through an employer where you or your spouse are actively working, provided that the employer has 20 or more employees.

I believe it is necessary to emphasize them here as well since much of the guidance regarding Medicare eligibility often gives the impression that everyone is obligated to sign up as soon as they turn 65, which is not necessarily the case. With that being said, the following sections will focus on qualifying for Medicare at the age of 65, even if you choose not to enroll at that time.

Meeting the requirements for Parts A, B, and D

As one would anticipate, the various components of Medicare have distinct eligibility requirements, coverage criteria, and costs. In the subsequent sections, you will find checklists outlining the conditions that must be fulfilled to qualify for Part A (hospital insurance), Part B (medical insurance), and Part D (prescription drug coverage) at the age of 65.

Even if you are not eligible for premium-free Part A, it is possible to meet the requirements for Part B and Part D coverage at the age of 65. Therefore, it is crucial to ensure timely enrollment for these parties to avoid incurring permanent late penalties.

Part A

You must be a citizen of the United States or a legal permanent resident (holder of a green card) and satisfy at least one of the following requirements to be eligible for Part A benefits (without paying premiums) at the age of 65 or older:

- By paying payroll taxes throughout your employment experience, you have accrued 40 credits, making you eligible for Social Security or railroad retirement benefits. Even if you are not currently receiving retirement benefits, you should still refer to the section titled "Qualifying for Part A on your own work record" for more information on the work record requirements.
- You are eligible based on your spouse's employment history, or under certain conditions, the employment history of your divorced or deceased spouse. This is described in the section titled "Being Eligible for Part A on Someone Else's Work Record."

If you are 65 or older and a citizen or authorized resident of the United States who has resided here for at least five years prior to qualifying for Medicare, you can qualify for Part A benefits without having 40 work credits. However, the following conditions must be met:

- You must enroll in both Parts A and B (further information in the section below).
- You must pay the entire Part A premium (which will be $458 per month in 2020) if you have 0 to 29 work credits.
- You or your spouse will pay a portion of the Part A premium ($252 per month in 2020) if you or they have 30 to 39 work credits.

Part B

If you are 65 years old or older, a U.S. citizen, or a legal resident (green-card holder) who has resided in the United States for a minimum of five years, you are eligible to receive Part

B benefits. To qualify, you must be enrolled in Part B, and one of the following conditions must apply:

- You pay a monthly premium, which can be the standard Part B premium ($144.60 per month in 2020) or a higher amount if your income exceeds a certain threshold that requires an income-related surcharge.
- Your state covers your Part B premium.

Part C

If you are 65 years of age or older, you could receive Part D benefits under the following circumstances:

- You are enrolled in Part A or Part B, or both.
- You enroll in either a stand-alone Part D drug plan or a Medicare Advantage plan that offers Medicare prescription drug coverage.
- One of the following conditions is applicable:
- You pay the monthly premium as required by your chosen plan.
- Your Part D plan premium is covered by the Extra Help program or a State Pharmacy Assistance Program.

Qualifying for Part A on your own work record

To be eligible for premium-free Part A benefits at the age of 65 or older, or to qualify for Social Security retirement benefits, you must earn 40 work credits, also known as quarters of coverage. Here's how these credits are calculated:

- Work credits are based on taxable income, specifically earnings on which you pay Social Security and Medicare payroll taxes. This includes wages from employer and earnings from self-employment. It does not include income from pensions, interest, dividends, or investments and savings.
- You need to earn a certain amount of money to receive one work credit, and this amount typically increases slightly each year. In 2020, the threshold was $1,410.
- The maximum number of work credits you can earn in a single year is four. In 2020, this would require earnings of $5,640. The timing of when you earn these credits does not matter. You can accumulate all four credits throughout the year, or you may earn them earlier within the first three months.
- Social Security will not credit the fourth credit, even if you earn all four before the end of the year, until October 1, the first day of the final quarter. To become completely insured and entitled for Part A benefits without monthly payments, for example, if you obtain your 40th credit in June, you must wait until October 1st.
- Accumulating 40 credits normally requires at least ten years of work, although these years do not have to be consecutive. Even though there are long stretches between

work periods, you still get credit whenever you put in time at the office and pay payroll taxes.

It's crucial to remember that not every job necessitates paying Social Security taxes. For instance, federal employees are not required to pay into Social Security and have access to their own retirement plan. All government employees must, however, pay Medicare payroll taxes since 1983 in order to get Part A benefits without premiums but not Social Security retirement benefits.

Different rules regarding work credits may apply in specific situations. If you are:

- Self-employed and earning less than $400 per year,
- Employed by a local or state government that opted out of Social Security participation,
- In the military (where additional credits may be granted in certain circumstances),
- Performing domestic work or farm work, or
- Working for a church or church organization that does not pay Social Security taxes, you should contact Social Security to discuss your specific credit requirements.

Being eligible for Part A on someone else's work record

If you have not accumulated enough work credits to qualify for Part A benefits without paying premiums, there is a possibility of qualifying based on the work record of your current or former spouse. However, it's important to note that the rules for eligibility vary depending on different circumstances.

Your spouse, current or past, has sufficient credit

If your current or former spouse has earned 40 work credits, you may qualify for premium-free Part A benefits based on their work record under the following circumstances:

- Current spouse: You have been married to your current spouse for at least one year, you are 65 years of age or older, and your spouse is at least 62 years old.
- Divorced spouse: You were married to your former spouse for at least ten years before the divorce was finalized, you have not remarried, you are 65 years of age or older, and your ex-spouse is at least 62 years old. (The remarriage status of your ex-spouse is not relevant in this case.)
- Deceased spouse: You were married to your late spouse for a minimum of nine months leading up to their death, you are 65 years of age or older, and you did not remarry before reaching age 60 (or age 50 if you are eligible for disability benefits).

- Divorced deceased spouse: You were married for at least ten years prior to the divorce, you did not remarry before reaching age 60 (or age 50 if you are eligible for disability benefits), and you are 65 years of age or older.

Neither you nor your spouse has 40 work credits

If your current or former spouse has fewer than 30 work credits, they do not contribute towards your eligibility for Medicare, which mcans you would still have to pay full premiums to receive Part A benefits. However, if your spouse has accumulated 30 to 39 work credits, you have the option to pay reduced Part A premiums based on their work record, even if you have no work credits yourself. This can have a significant financial impact. In 2020, the full Part A premium was $458 per month, while the reduced premium was $252 per month. It's worth noting that once your current or ex-spouse earns 40 work credits, you become eligible for Part A benefits on their work record without the need to pay premiums.

Combining your work credits with those of your spouse to qualify for premium-free Part A is not allowed. Even if you have some work credits and your spouse has more, you can only meet the criteria for paying a reduced Part A premium based on your spouse's credits. In other words, you cannot combine your credits to reach a total of 51 credits between the two of you.

You're the foreign spouse of a U.S. citizen or legal resident

Typically, individuals who are not U.S. citizens and have not worked in the United States must become permanent legal residents (green-card holders) and reside continuously in the country for at least five years to qualify for Medicare benefits.

However, there is an exception for green-card holders who are 65 or older and have been married to a U.S. citizen or legal resident for at least one year. If your spouse is age 62 or older and has earned 40 work credits, you are eligible for full Medicare benefits, including premium-free Part A, based on your spouse's work record. This eligibility does not require you to fulfill the five-year residency requirement.

You're in a same sex marriage

Following a landmark decision by the U.S. Supreme Court in June 2015, which established the constitutional right to same-sex marriage nationwide, couples in same-sex marriages are entitled to the same federal benefits as those in opposite-sex marriages. This includes the right for one same-sex spouse to qualify for full Medicare benefits without paying premiums for Part A, based on the work record of the other spouse, if all the eligibility criteria described in previous sections are met.

The Supreme Court's ruling occurred precisely two years after another historic decision that invalidated significant portions of the Defense of Marriage Act (DOMA). Enacted in

1996, this law defined a spouse as "a man or woman who is legally married to a person of the opposite sex," thereby denying numerous federal benefits to individuals legally married to someone of the same sex. However, the repeal of DOMA in 2013 did not immediately grant couples in states that prohibited same-sex marriage the right to qualify for premium-free Part A based on their spouse's work record. This was because, under a separate law, the Social Security Administration was obligated to adhere to the marriage laws of the state where individuals applying for Medicare resided, rather than where they were married. The Supreme Court's ruling in 2015 changed this situation, ensuring that same-sex spouses have equal rights to those of other married couples, regardless of their state of residence, including the 13 states that still prohibited same-sex marriage at the time of the decision.

You are unmarried but live in a domestic partnership

Typically, you cannot qualify for premium-free Part A benefits based on the work record of a domestic partner with whom you are not legally married, regardless of whether your partner is of the same sex or opposite sex, or whether you have been covered by their employer's health insurance.

For individuals in domestic partnerships who are covered by their partner's employer health plan, it is important to familiarize yourself with the regulations concerning enrollment in Medicare Part B.

Qualifying for Medicare under Age 65 on the Basis of Disability

Individuals with disabilities have often faced challenges in securing affordable health insurance due to their medical conditions. However, Medicare helps by providing coverage for three specific groups of disabled individuals:

1. Those who have been receiving Social Security disability payments for a minimum of two years.
2. Those with permanent kidney failure, also known as End-Stage Renal Disease (ESRD).
3. Those diagnosed with Lou Gehrig's disease, medically known as amyotrophic lateral sclerosis (ALS).

In the subsequent sections, I will elaborate on the qualification process for Medicare if you belong to any of these categories.

Receiving disability payments

If you are unable to earn above a specific monthly income due to an illness, injury, or disability that is expected to last for at least one year, you may meet the eligibility criteria for Social Security Disability Insurance (SSDI). To obtain information on eligibility and application procedures, you can contact Social Security at 800-772-1213 or the TTY number 800-325-0778.

Once your application has been reviewed by Social Security, they will inform you about your eligibility for SSDI. If approved, you will start receiving monthly cash payments, commencing five months after the determined onset date of your disability.

Eventually, you will also become eligible for Medicare benefits that are identical to those provided to individuals aged 65 and older. However, there is a requirement to wait for 24 months as per the law before your Medicare coverage begins.

The subsequent sections provide answers to common inquiries regarding Medicare for individuals receiving disability payments.

How does the 24-month waiting period work?

In most cases, Medicare coverage typically starts on the first day of the 25th month of receiving SSDI payments. This 25th month is considered the fourth month of your initial enrollment period. It's important to note that you don't need to actively apply for Medicare.

Once you begin receiving SSDI, Social Security automatically enrolls you in Part A and Part B. Your Medicare card will be sent to you via mail around two or three months before your coverage becomes effective. However, if you wish to opt out of Part B, it is possible to do so. Nevertheless, it's important to be aware of potential pitfalls associated with this decision.

In certain circumstances, the waiting period for Medicare may be shorter than two years. For instance, if you initially apply for SSDI and your application is denied, you have the option to file an appeal. If you succeed in the appeal, Social Security will retroactively approve your application to the first month when you should have been eligible for SSDI. As a result, the 24-month waiting period for Medicare would commence from that earlier date, which could be many months or even years prior to when you begin receiving SSDI payments.

Note: The 24-month waiting period for Medicare does not have to be continuous. This means that if you received SSDI for a certain number of months and later became ineligible, but then qualified for SSDI again later, even if it's years later, all the months you previously received SSDI will be collectively counted towards the 24-month waiting period for Medicare.

If you have not received your Medicare card by the 23rd month of receiving SSDI, it is recommended to contact Social Security at 800-772-1213 or the TTY number 800-325-0778 to inquire if there might be any issues or complications.

How long does Medicare coverage last?

If you qualify for Medicare through disability, your Medicare benefits will remain in effect if you receive SSDI payments and potentially even longer. If you return to work and lose SSDI, under certain circumstances and based on your income level, your Medicare benefits can continue for an additional 93 months (eight and a half years). If your employer provides health benefits, you are required to enroll in them, and Medicare will then serve as secondary insurance. However, if the employer's health insurance includes a health savings account, you may not be able to utilize it. After the 93-month period, if you continue to have disabilities and are employed, you can maintain your Medicare benefits. However, you will need to pay a monthly premium for Part A services and for Part B, unless you qualify for assistance through a Medicare Savings Program offered by your state.

If you are already enrolled in Medicare when you turn 65, your coverage will seamlessly continue. However, at that point, your eligibility for Medicare will be based on your age rather than disability. During this transition, you don't need to take any action. However, you will have another seven-month initial enrollment period, which begins three months before you turn 65. During this period, you could:

- Explore better options for Medigap supplemental insurance, which may have been unaffordable or denied to you when you were under 65
- Make changes to your Medicare coverage choices if you wish to do so.
- Stop paying any late enrollment penalties that you may have incurred earlier.

Does railroad retirement disability work in the same way?

If you are insured under the railroad retirement system instead of Social Security and have disabilities, the rules differ based on the classification of your disability. Here are the variations:

- Total Disability: If you have total disability, meaning you are unable to work in any job, you become eligible for Medicare coverage after receiving disability payments for 24 months.
- Occupational Disability: If you have occupational disability, meaning you are unable to perform your regular railroad job but may still be capable of working in another capacity, you do not qualify for early Medicare benefits before the age of 65. However, if you are granted a disability freeze at some point due to a severe medical condition that prevents you from engaging in any work or because you are 55 years of age or older and blind, you will become eligible for Medicare 29 weeks after the freeze period begins.

Suffering from permanent kidney failure (ESRD)

End-stage renal disease (ESRD) is a chronic medical condition characterized by permanent kidney failure. It requires regular dialysis or a kidney transplant to maintain proper kidney function. In Medicare, ESRD is considered a specific condition with unique coverage rules. Unlike other situations, there is no waiting period for Medicare coverage if you have ESRD, but certain conditions must be met. These conditions are as follows:

1. Full insurance: You must be fully insured, which means you have earned 40 work credits from your own work record to qualify for Social Security or railroad retirement benefits. Alternatively, you may have worked as a government employee who qualified for Medicare through payroll taxes. Please refer to the earlier section titled "Qualifying for Part A on your own work record" for more details.

2. Spouse or dependent child: You can also qualify for Medicare if you are the spouse or dependent child of a person who is fully insured.

3. The start of Medicare coverage depends on the type of care you require (dialysis or transplant) and whether you have coverage under an employer plan. If you receive Medicare solely based on having ESRD, your coverage continues for 12 months after you stop dialysis or 36 months after you've had a kidney transplant and no longer need dialysis. However, if you need to resume dialysis or undergo another transplant, Medicare coverage begins again without any waiting period.

ALS, also known as Amyotrophic lateral sclerosis or Lou Gehrig's disease, is a degenerative condition that affects the nerve cells in the brain and spinal cord, leading to muscle deterioration and loss of movement. In 2001, Congress passed a law that eliminates the 24-month waiting period for Medicare coverage for individuals diagnosed with ALS.

To qualify for Medicare if you have ALS, you must go through the standard process of being approved for Social Security or railroad retirement disability benefits. Medicare coverage starts on the first day of the month when your disability benefit payments begin.

Falling through the Cracks: Health-Care Options if You Can't Get Medicare Yet

In the complex and fragmented American healthcare system, some individuals inevitably fall through the cracks. Consider the following scenarios:

1. If you're under 65 and have qualified for disability payments, you may have to wait for up to two years before becoming eligible for Medicare coverage.

2. If you're 65 or older but haven't lived in the United States for the required five years as a legal immigrant, you may not yet qualify for Medicare.

3. If you're nearing Medicare eligibility but have lost or never had a job with health benefits, and you're in poor health, you may be concerned about accessing healthcare.
4. If your spouse, who provides your health insurance through their employment, is older than you and is retiring, leaving both of you without employer benefits, you may wonder about your healthcare options while your spouse joins Medicare.

In any of these situations, it's important to explore and consider potential avenues for healthcare coverage while waiting for Medicare. The following sections provide information on possibilities to explore, although it's worth noting that not all options may be available to everyone.

If you can acquire it, nice work: securing a position with benefits

If you or your spouse are able to access one, having a job with health insurance is often the best choice. Regardless of age, health status, or pre-existing medical issues, firms with 20 or more employees are required to offer all employees the same health insurance benefits, including coverage for spouses.

But what if you're younger than your spouse, don't have employer insurance, and your partner is thinking about retiring? Some businesses may continue to offer insurance for a younger spouse after the employee retires, either by extending retiree benefits that cover both people or until the younger spouse reaches Medicare age. Unfortunately, this younger spouse frequently lacks insurance. If this applies to you,

Paying for COBRA temporary insurance

In accordance with the Consolidated Omnibus Budget Reconciliation Act of 1986 (COBRA), those who have quit their jobs or lost their jobs are still eligible for up to 18 months of health insurance via their previous employer. However, they are obligated to pay the full premiums, which includes the employer's part, which may be expensive. The COBRA coverage is still available to the qualifying spouses and dependent children of departing employees, even if they do not choose it themselves.

Your COBRA benefits will expire if you decide to enroll in COBRA and then become eligible for Medicare. Your spouse, however, might then be qualified for an additional 36 months of COBRA coverage.

There are additional statutes in some jurisdictions that provide COBRA coverage for longer periods of time. if you were previously a Medicare beneficiary.

Buying Individual Insurance with the help of Online Marketplace

According to the 2010 Affordable Care Act which is also regarded as Obamacare or you can also call it ACA, enables uninsured individuals to purchase private health insurance through government owned or private insurance exchanges called the "Marketplace." This law brought a significant change, allowing people to buy the health insurance on the individual level basis which can be regardless of the health status or with the pre-existing medical conditions since the year 2014. As a result, millions of previously uninsured individuals now have access to coverage.

Please note that the information provided here is current unless the ACA is repealed.

If you do not have health insurance through an employer or government programs like Medicare and Medicaid, you can utilize the online Marketplace, which serves as a one-stop platform for comparing and selecting various health care plans, prescription drugs, screenings, tests, vaccinations, and mental health services.

Insurance companies selling plans through the Marketplace can charge higher premiums based on age, and they can also impose surcharges of up to 50 percent for smokers. However, they cannot deny or limit coverage or charge higher premiums based on past or present health conditions. Furthermore, they are prohibited from imposing annual or lifetime dollar limits on coverage.

Can you have Marketplace insurance in addition to Medicare? In most cases, no. Insurers are prohibited from selling plans to individuals with Medicare, and even if it were possible, you would not qualify for subsidies. However, it may be possible to choose a Marketplace plan instead of Medicare if you would have to pay premiums for Part A. It's important to be cautious, though, as failing to enroll in Medicare Parts A and B when required may result in late penalties.

Open enrollment for Marketplace insurance typically occurs from November 1 to December 15 in most states. However, California, Colorado, and Washington, DC, have permanently extended their open enrollment periods, and Pennsylvania's new state-run exchange has extended open enrollment through January 15, 2021. State-run exchanges have the flexibility to make the open enrollment period longer.

Special enrollment periods (SEPs) are available for signing up with a plan during other times of the year under specific circumstances. These circumstances include losing other insurance, getting married or divorced, adding a child to the family, gaining citizenship, becoming a lawful resident of the United States, being released from prison, or moving out of your plan's service area. The SEP generally lasts for up to 60 days following these events.

Beginning in January 2019, the ACA no longer imposes a federal tax penalty for individuals who choose not to have health insurance coverage. However, it's important to note that some states still enforce their own penalties. If you have employer coverage, Medicaid, or Medicare Part A, you are considered to have comparable coverage and are not required to purchase additional health insurance. Therefore, you will not face any penalties. However, it's worth mentioning that having only Medicare Part B does not qualify as comparable coverage and may result in tax penalties.

Necessitating the buying of health insurance out of the Obamacare Marketplace

Considering the uncertain future of Obamacare and the lack of knowledge regarding its potential replacement, it is worthwhile to explore the option of purchasing individual health insurance on the open market. Prior to the implementation of the main provisions of the Affordable Care Act in 2014, many individuals without employer insurance obtained coverage in this manner.

During the pre-ACA era, individuals aged 50 and above often encountered difficulties in obtaining health insurance, and if they did find coverage, it was typically expensive. This was because insurance companies were legally allowed to deny coverage or charge higher premiums based on existing or pre-existing medical conditions.

However, there was one previous law in place, HIPAA (Health Insurance Portability and Accountability Act of 1996), that provided limited protections to certain individuals seeking individual insurance policies for themselves or their families. According to HIPAA, an individual has the right to buy insurance that does not exclude or limit coverage for pre-existing medical issues provided they have had group or COBRA insurance for at least 18 months. Nonetheless, it is important to note that this coverage may still come at a high cost and does not include the government subsidies provided by the ACA to help reduce premiums.

Getting health care without insurance

Icon TIP If you are unable to afford insurance and do not meet the eligibility requirements for assistance, there is still a possibility of receiving medical care through community clinics that offer services to uninsured individuals either for free, at a low cost, or based on your ability to pay.

Chapter 6
How to Enroll in Medicare and What to Expect

Topics:

- ➢ Understanding how to join both Parts A and B of Medicare Automatically
- ➢ Understanding signing up in Medicare Parts A and B from inside and outside the US
- ➢ Learning when and how to decline Medicare Parts A and B coverage.
- ➢ Ensuring you fully understand when your coverage takes effect.
- ➢ Understanding the transition from the Obamacare to conventional Medicare

You can save yourself by knowing the process and when to enroll for Medicare from unwelcome surprises like late penalties. While most people dread this part, signing up for Medicare is a straightforward process. (Did I just hear an exhale of relief?)

This chapter takes you through the nitty gritty of signing up in Part A and B (traditional Medicare), except for Part D aka Medicare Advantage Plans. To sign up for Medicare MA plan, you should first enroll for Parts A and B. Once you have Part A and B, you are eligible for a Part D prescription drug plan. Enrolling in Part D Medicare or MA comes with its fair share of complexities as you will have to go through heaps of private and personalized plans accessible in your vicinity and then choose only one - Believe me, that is a next-level ballgame.

Here we have shortlisted three simple ways to plunge inside the Medicare worldliness as per your situation:

- Automatically sign up if you are collecting disability benefits already, have retired from railroad, or Social Security.
- Promptly apply for admission within the US if you are still to draw these advantages.
- Enroll if you are an overseas.

In this chapter, you will also learn the process of opting out of Medicare Part A and B Plans if wanting to and the reasons you should be careful about doing so. Furthermore, we have discussed when your coverage will take effect, depending on your signup date. And lastly, the technicalities and the processes of switching from the Obamacare to Medicare - a shift affecting plethora of people daily.

The A and B Supplements to Medicare The Social Security Administration, not Medicare, is responsible for the enrollment and disenrollment procedures. Hence, if you want to sign up or opt-out, contact a federal official, Social Security.

Having Your Medicare Parts A and B Enrollment Handled Automatically

As mentioned previously, there is an advantage of Social Security, that it enrolls you automatically in the following circumstances:

- You are about to turn 65 and have already been collecting retirement benefits from Railroad Retirement Road or Social Security.
- You are below 65 but eligible due to disability.
- If you have crossed 65 and have been procrastinating on the enrollment process because you have been covered under your partner's (husband/wife) active employment you may contact the Social Security or Railway Retirement Board to draw payouts from retirement benefits.

Note: If you get railway and Social Security benefits but reside outside the United States, you will not be immediately eligible for Medicare. If you are a Puerto Rican resident and have begun receiving these payments, you will automatically be enrolled in Part A. Part B enrollment may still be required, however.

If the first and following circumstances happen to be with you, you will receive a Medicare ID card from Social Security just three months prior to when your insurance takes effect. In the last situation, Social Security first approves your retirement benefits then you will receive the Medicare ID card. In case of delay, dial 800-772 -1213 and TTY 800 - 325 -0778.

The blue, red, and white cards of Medicare are your passport to healthcare facilities. Once you have signed up for it, make sure to collect every envelope sent to you by Social Security Administration. When your mailbox is filled with unwanted private insurance offers, it can be tempting to toss them all away, but it's important to be careful. So, look out for the Social Security Administration logo on the left-hand corner of the envelopes.

The white-colored envelope contains your Medicare ID card and a letter stating the date your coverage will take effect. Your ID card also has the dates printed from when you can begin availing of Medicare benefits. For instance, if you are turning 65 on June 15, your card should arrive in March with the letter letting you know you that your Parts A and B insurance will be effective on June 1.

If for any reason you want to opt out of Part A or B, you can refer to the Social Security envelope enclosing your Medicare card ID card for details on how to withdraw from Part A or B within a certain deadline. That said, you need to diligently think about your decision before acting it out, as in some situations, it may not be what you should do. We have dedicated an entire section to address whether you should opt out of Part A or B. So, make sure you stop by that section before moving forward.

Count Me In! Procedures for Obtaining Medicare Parts A and B

Back when Social Security's full retirement age was 65, many Americans stop working at that age and were eligible for Medicare benefits. They might apply for Medicare, railway and Social Security benefits simultaneously by simply strolling over to the local Social Security office. Unfortunately, this is no longer the case.

The entire retirement plan has been delayed by a few months annually for the last several years, even though Medicare enrollment is still available for persons aged 65 and higher. Full retirement age is now 67 for anybody born in 1960 or later. They may begin taking a portion of their benefits at age 62, but won't get the entire amount until they reach age 67. Therefore, as previously indicated, they will not be automatically enrolled in Medicare.

To Register Within the United States

It's no surprise that Americans have an easier time applying for Medicare benefits than those from other countries. However, you should be familiar with the specifics of the three application options available to you, such as what to do if you leave the nation or state for a portion of the year. In addition, if English is not your first language, you may need to take further measures to guarantee your comprehension of the enrolling procedure. Below, you'll find comprehensive coverage of all three of these issues:

Signing Up when you are Overseas

There are three enrollment periods for Medicare Part A and/or B: the initial enrollment period, which begins when you turn 65, the special enrollment period, which begins when you turn 70, and the annual general enrollment period, which begins on January 1 and ends on March 31 of each year if you missed enrolling during the initial enrollment period or the special enrollment period. The specifics of these sign-up windows are covered in further depth below.

If you opt to apply via phone, you will require to mail all your original documents or leave them at your nearby office of Social Security. However, if you want to or prioritize to have those documents with you and keep them from going out of sight, you can take them to the office and bring them afterward. Social Security prohibits sending off your foreign birth certificate, immigration documents, or any proof of permanent residencies, such as a Green Card, as they are vital documents and are hard to retrieve if lost.

Online applying is the easiest method of enrolling in Medicare as it hardly takes ten minutes of your time. For some, it may not be the best course of action, and the in-person method may prove to be effective.

- If you got enrolled in Part A when you were 65 years or older, during a special enrollment period, and you sign up for Part B after losing work or employer-based insurance, you won't be able to apply online.
- If you are out of the US, you will not be able to apply online. (We have explained that in the later section in detail.)
- If your case is complicated, you may not be able to apply online due to the challenges you may face online. In such cases, Social Security reaches out to guide you through the process.
- If you are not comfortable mailing crucial documents like your birth certificate, marriage certificate, or immigration documents, you can bring them to the office of Social Security with you instead.
- Walking down to a local Social Security office can assist you explain the reason you are not enrolling in Part B of Medicare during the first enrollment period if you choose to do so because you already have employer-based insurance and prefer to enroll in Part A during the initial enrollment period. Make sure to document the reason you have not signed up for Part B in your computer records and cross-check if you are complying with the rules.
- If you continue to work past age 65, but your company's insurance provides you with a health saving account, enrolling in Medicare will stop you from contributing to your saving account. So just tapping the 'submit' option on the website will cause you some serious troubles.
- If you want consultation regarding when the best time is to enroll in Medicare and which is the easiest process to do so, an in-person application would be your best bet.

Once you have opted for a method per your convenience, Social Security will dispatch a printout stating your registration information that has been added to your data. The printout will help cross-check if all the information has been entered correctly and get it fixed if not. If you have any missing information in your application, in that case, Social Security will contact you itself for adjustments.

When dialing Social Security, be prepared to be put on hold for a while until the operator connects you to a customer representative, which takes roughly around 45 minutes or more. Social Security facilitates tons of customers daily, with 10,000 people turning 65 each year and others for general queries. So be patient and plan to keep a puzzle or a cube in your hand to keep yourself busy while you wait.

Retirees Moving in Different States All Year

Most retired people in America are seagulls and travel to different places in the country during parts of the year. Others drive to different states to visit their family and friends for festivals. A small chunk of them makes recreational vehicles their home and are on the move all year round. Considering any circumstance out of these, how would they enroll in Medicare?

Social Security requires one permanent residence, also called principal residence, to sign up for Medicare. Any state where you are registered to vote, file taxes, get your driving license, and so is considered your principal residence. Even if you are on the move in your RV all year round, you will still sign up for Medicare using your principal residence.

If you are homeless and do not own any place of your own, Social Security may use your shelter's address and number, or any place you can collect your mails or parcels. For further queries in this regard, you may contact Social Security at 800-772-1213 (TTY 800-325-0778).

While Medicare requires the candidate to sign up in one place, they can avail of all the benefits nationwide - enabling them decide right about the type of insurance they select.

Understanding Medicare Application Jargon

Whether English is your first language or not, comprehending the jargon used in Medicare applications may be intimidating to the candidates. So, when applying for Medicare, don't shy away from asking for assistance or help, and ensure you fully get the idea of what are you signing up for.

When visiting or dialing to Social Security office, you can always ask for an interpreter to help you out. They can speak and interpret over 150 languages and will assist you for no additional cost. To request interpreter services, you may follow these instructions:

1. Dial the main Social Security number listed previously. An IVR (Interactive voice response) will tell you to dial 1 for instructions in English and 2 for instructions in Spanish. Dial your desired number, and you will be instructed in your chosen language. For a third language, press 1.
2. Next, when the IVR asks how they can help, say 'operator.'
3. A customer representative will be connected to you shortly, say, 'I need an interpreter.'

You will be asked to wait for a bit until you are connected to an interpreter. He/she will then act as a translator between you and the official. The same service is available for in-person applications as well. And of course, if you know a little English, you can get help from a friend or a family member to get you through the process. They will be required to share your SSN while making the call.

Overseas Americans are provided with certain options to enroll in Medicare. The procedure of enrolling, as well as any penalties for late enrollment, may vary depending on whether you apply during your personal enrollment window while remaining overseas or after you return to the US. The following section will take you through the application process for Medicare while living abroad.

Medicare Enrolment

How to Sign up if you are Fully Insured for Benefits of Medicare?

One can be eligible for full Medicare pluses if they or their spouse have enough work credits with paid payroll taxes. Simply put, you will be eligible for Part A benefits if you fulfill the above requirements at no additional cost.

How to Enroll if There is no Entirely Insured Medicare Benefits?

You can qualify for Medicare premium-free Part A benefits even if you don't possess optimum work pluses on your record. Part A benefits typically include hospital stays and require monthly premiums to avail themselves of the benefits. You can't buy into the Plan while your permanent address is registered outside the US.

Whether you own a property, have a telephone number, or have a family living in the US, you can't buy into Medicare Part A until you reside permanently in the States under Social Security Guidelines. According to the rules, a candidate cannot simultaneously establish residencies in two countries.

No of how long the person has lived abroad or how long it has been since they turned 65, they will be eligible for an initial enrollment period to purchase Part A and sign up for B at no extra cost. Returning international students have from the beginning of the month they get home until the end of the third month to register in classes. Your first enrollment period, for instance, will go through November 30 if you return in August. Your first day of coverage under the Plan will be the first of the next calendar month after you enroll. If you miss out on enrolling at that time, the next general enrollment period begins on January 1 and runs through March 31. Please be aware that there may be permanent late fines if you do not have coverage in place by July 1.

After the applicant has arrived in the United States, he may register in Part A and Part B by calling the Social Security Administration at 800-772-1213.

Medicare Enrollment from outside the US

For queries regarding Medicare enrollment, it is advisable to reach out to Social Security Administration. However, note that you cannot directly dial its main toll-free number while living outside the US. Instead, it is suggested to contact them via mail or phone. In all circumstances, make sure to provide your details correctly, including your full name, home address, contact number, also number of Social Security.

How You May Contact SSA by Mail:

If you opt to contact Social Security Administration by mail, write to their Office of Earnings and International Operations, P.O Box 17775, Baltimore, MD, 21235, USA.

How to Contact SSA by Phone:

Overseas may contact the Social Security Administration at 410-965-0160. However, note that you will be required to pay the calling fee as Social Security doesn't give access a toll-free dial for overseas calls. Also, you must call during US business hours in the time zone of easter.

Refusing to Participate in Medicare Parts A and B

Whether or whether you should cancel your Medicare Part A or Part B coverage is a personal decision. But there's always something to think about before making a final decision, so you don't waste money on unnecessary missteps.

When you become eligible for Social Security or disability benefits, Social Security will automatically register you in Medicare Parts A and B unless you opt out. You will get a letter in the mail giving you the choice to opt out of Part B. If you change your mind, you may cancel at any time. If, on the other hand, you are not receiving disability or retirement benefits and must enroll in Parts A and B independently, you have the freedom to choose whether or not to do so.

Next up, we have detailed the pitfalls and possibilities for deciding not to opt for Part A and B when you sign up. We have further explained how to withdraw from Part B when you are already enrolled in it.

Declining Part A

You cannot decline Medicare Part A if you are collecting disability and retirement benefits. However, there are two ways to opt out of Part A: withdraw your application for disability and retirement benefits simultaneously or repay the government if you have already collected all the payouts. This sounds like a burdensome task and has already been subjected to a lawsuit against the US government. Declining Part A is quite rare among Americans after all; why would anyone want to give up on the benefits they had been paying for with their tax money?

You may be eligible to decline Medicare Part A if you have employer-provided health insurance with a high deductible and a health savings account funded with pre-tax dollars and you continue to work past the Medicare eligibility period. There are, however, limitations to this approach. For example, Medicare takes over as the major healthcare insurance payer for businesses with less than 20 workers, so your business must have at least that many people working for it. Next, it has already been established that health savings account contributions must be stopped once Medicare coverage begins. The money in your HSA, however, may be used to cover eligible medical expenditures.

If you are eligible for Part A at no additional cost, you won't be hit with a late penalty for delayed enrollment in Part A. If you are qualified to join Medicare by paying premiums for Part A but you wait until after the deadline has passed, you may be subject to late fines. Note that once enrolled in Part A, you can only opt-out within the next 12 months.

Opting out of part B

If you are considering opting out of Medicare Part B, we suggest you rethink your decision, even though you must pay a monthly premium. (Individuals with limited income and resources are eligible to receive help from Medicare to pay premiums through Medicare Savings Program. Whether to opt-out of Part B coverage is an important decision, especially when you are signed up automatically. Hence, you must be careful about how to deal with it as per your situation.

Next up, we have discussed when it is okay to opt out of Part B coverage. In other terms, when it is the right time to opt out, it doesn't cost you money or make you regret it in the future. Strangely, Medicare has different rules for people who have Medicare because they have reached 65 or more and those who have it early due to disability. Let's look at each group separately to learn when the right time is for each of them to decline Part B coverage. Then we will discuss when it's risky for each group to decline Part B coverage.

Disenrolling from Part B

Part B should be declined at age 65 only if you or your spouse are covered by employer-sponsored health insurance that covers medical bills in full before Medicare does. In such a situation, you won't be penalized for late enrollment in Part B coverage. So, if you are not already collecting retirement and Social Security benefits, you can avoid signing up for Part B. On the other hand, if you have already been enrolled in Part B because you have been collecting those benefits, in that case, you can follow the instructions provided in the Social Security letter to decline Part B coverage under the give timeline. (Check the earlier section "How to Get Automatically Enrolled in Medicare Part A and B" for more information on this)

If you decide to opt out of Part B, you will no longer be responsible for paying the associated premium. The premium might be withdrawn automatically from your Social Security or retirement check. It also guarantees your right to purchase Medigap insurance as a retiree, with all government safeguards in place. When obtained at certain periods within six months of enrolling in Part B coverage, this will prevent insurance carriers from refusing to sell you Medigap and from charging you rates based on your health condition. This benefit is forfeited if you resign within six months of turning 65 and enrolling in Medicare Part B.

If both you and your spouse are employed by the same employer, you are eligible for a special enrollment period and may put off signing up for Medicare Part B, just like any other married couple. Domestic spouses of any sexual orientation are exempt from this provision.

Learning When to Decline Medicare Part B Coverage under 65

Following are the situations under which you should not accept Medicare Part B coverage:

- You or your spouse are covered by health insurance via your employer, provided that the business has 100 or more full-time workers.
- If your employer has 100 or more workers, you likely qualify for group health insurance via your employer.

In this context, "family members" refers to anybody who, regardless of marital status, is considered to be domestically related to the employee and so eligible for health care under the insurance plan.

Getting to Know - Not Accepting Medicare Part B Might Be Risky At Any Age

Whether you qualify for Medicare because of age or disability, if you have health insurance that will become secondary to Medicare, you should never decline Part B. The contents are as follows:

- Health insurance that you obtain by yourself and not your employer from an open insurance market.
- Employer-provided health insurance with less than 20 employees. (For age 65 or older)
- Employer-provided health insurance with less than 100 employees. (For those with Medicare due to disability)
- COBRA or retiree benefits from a previous employer you or your spouse worked for
- Military-provided health benefits under TRICARE for Life retiree program.

When determining whether or not to participate in Medicare Part B, it's important to give serious consideration to your unique situation. If you are eligible for Medicare Part B, you should strongly consider enrolling in it due to the substantial benefits it provides. When Medicare is the main payer, it covers medical costs before any other sources. However, there is a genuine danger of having a claim that Medicare would have paid for rejected if you choose to forgo Part B coverage. It's possible that you'll have to foot the full amount alone. In the worst case scenario, you might be compelled to repay any funds spent on healthcare services rendered since you became Medicare-eligible if your insurer fails to timely notify you that you are not enrolled in Medicare Part B.

Not everyone is like this, however. For those already insured under the Federal Employee Health Benefits Program, enrollment in Medicare Part B is unnecessary. Medicare's relationship with complementary health insurance programs is explored in the following chapters. In addition, not all businesses with less than 20 workers need their eligible employees to enroll in Medicare.

Conclusively, to decide whether to accept or decline Medicare Plan B, you first need to determine if they are primary or secondary payers to your other insurance plans.

Knowing When Your Coverage Begins

Knowing the time of your coverage can help you save a generous amount of energy. Knowledge of your enrollment timings can help you take several right decisions. For instance, signing up on time is a great benefit of knowing when your coverage begins, but how? Knowing that you can only sign up during the general enrollment period in January and that your coverage will begin in July of the following year if you miss your personal enrollment deadline can encourage you to enroll on time.

Consider this scenario instead: Picture yourself working for a company that provided health insurance until you turned 65. Now, your employer is offering remarkable retiree health benefits that will cover you for life. It's a rare and fortunate situation because retiree benefits are never guaranteed. To be safe, you enroll in Medicare Part B, but you put off paying the monthly payment for as long as you can. You may save a lot of money on Medicare Part B premiums in the near term and avoid late penalties by waiting until the conclusion of the eight-month special enrollment period that retirees are eligible to.

You have several options for signing up for Part A and Part B, depending on your situation. Here are the different time frames available:

1. Initial Enrollment Period (IEP): To calculate your Medicare eligibility, add seven months to the month in which you turn 65 or become disabled. During this time, you may enroll in both Part A and Part B.
2. Special Enrollment Period (SEP): You are eligible for an eight-month SEP if you or your spouse leave a job that provides health insurance after age 65. Parts A and B enrollment is open at this time.
3. General Enrollment Period (GEP): The GEP runs from January 1 to March 31 each year. If you miss the deadline for your IEP or SEP, you can use this three-month period to enroll in Part A and Part B.

Refer to Table 7-1 for a detailed overview of when your coverage will begin based on the enrollment periods mentioned above. This table only applies to those who opt for Medicare Parts A and B and not to those who are automatically enrolled.

TABLE 7-1

Enrollment Situation IEP/ When You Turn 65	**Coverage Begins**
Initial 3 months of your Initial Enrollment Period (IEP)	When you turn 65, which might bc the first of the month in which you turn 65, or the first of the month before if your birthday is on the first of the month.
The 4th month of your IEP	The first of the next month
The 5th month of your IEP	As of the beginning of the second month after your registration
The 6th month of your IEP	On the first of the third month after signing up
The 7th month of your IEP	Your enrolment will begin on the first day of the third month.
Special Enrollment Period (SEP) - Covered over 65 by Insurance from a Current Employer	
Any time while you have this coverage, provided that your IEP has expired	The first day of the month after you enroll
During the 8-month SEP after active employment or insurance ends (whichever comes first)	The first day of the month after you enroll
Outside IEP/SEP	
General Enrollment Period (GEP)	The following July 1

Table 7-1 provides an overview of the broader aspects. It highlights the simplicity of the special and general enrollment sessions. Your coverage will begin on the first of the month after your enrollment if you are eligible for a Special Enrollment Period (SEP). However, if you miss the deadline and have to enroll during a General Enrollment Period (GEP), your coverage won't start until July of the following year.

When you enroll in the first quarter of your Individualized Education Program

However, starting coverage during your Initial Enrollment Period (IEP) is a little more complicated and requires additional information.

Important for enrolling in Medicare, the Initial Enrollment Period (IEP) lasts for seven months. However, as detailed below, your coverage won't start until the following month if you join in the middle of the year. In addition, I'll describe what happens if you're under 65 years old and your Medicare coverage is reinstated retroactively as a result of an appeal.

If you sign up during the first three months of your IEP, your 65th birthday will likely fall inside the fourth month, the middle of your seven-month term. Your coverage will begin as soon as feasible if you enroll in Medicare Parts A and B within the first three months after turning 65, often on the first day of the month in which you turn 65.

Nonetheless, if your 65th birthday falls precisely on the first day of a given month, your initial enrollment period is adjusted, resulting in your coverage starting on the first day of the preceding month.

It's worth noting that this regulation is often unfamiliar to many regular Medicare beneficiaries. If, however, your birthday falls on the first of the month, this is really important information for you to have. To further understand IEP enrollments, consider the following:

- Since Hannah's 65th birthday was on April 29, her first membership term was from January 1 to July 31 (a span of seven months). Her effective start date for coverage was April 1 as she enrolled within the first three months of her IEP (January through March).
- John, on the other hand, was born on September 1. As a result, the dates of his Individualized Education Program (IEP) were changed from June 1 to December 31 to May 1 to November 30. If he signed up in May, June, or July, his coverage wouldn't start until August 1st, a full month before his actual birthday.

When you sign up during IEP months four through seven

Your coverage will be delayed if you do not enroll during the first three months of your Initial Enrollment Period (IEP). Early enrollment is rewarded by Medicare. Delays are described below according to enrollment month:

- During the fourth month, coverage will not commence until the first day of the following month.
- There is a two-month lag between the fifth month payment and the start of coverage.
- If you sign up in the sixth month, you won't be covered until the start of the ninth month (a three-month wait).
- If you sign up in the seventh month, you won't be covered until the tenth (a three-month wait) of the year.

Let's take Bren, for example, who will be 65 on June 20. His IEP has a duration of seven months, from March 1st to September 30th. Signing up in March, April, or May will have him covered beginning on June 1. However, the following delays will occur if he enrolls in subsequent months:

- If your birthday is in June, your coverage will begin on July 1.
- There is a two-month lag between July (the fifth IEP month) and the start of coverage (September 1).
- Coverage commences on November 1 (after a three-month delay) in the month of August (the sixth IEP month).
- Coverage starts on December 1 (after a three-month delay) in the month of September (the seventh IEP month).

Please keep in mind that December 1 is regarded as the commencement of Medicare coverage when calculating these delays.

Chapter 7
Making Sense of Medicare's Many Options

Topics:

- Acknowledging that your first choice determines later ones.
- Grasping the differences between traditional Medicare and Medicare Advantage plans.
- Understanding the differences between Medigap and Medicare Advantage

Politicians' repeated, oversimplified, "one-size-fits-all" descriptions of Medicare are a source of sarcastic amusement for me. Employing such clichéd rhetoric reveals a glaring ignorance of the program's intricate workings. Just picture a Medicare that genuinely adhered to this uniformity; it would undoubtedly be a far more streamlined and comprehensible system, rendering lengthy explanations unnecessary. Alas, that is not the case, for Medicare presents a multitude of diverse options. Yet, this vast array of choices often leaves individuals bewildered and overwhelmed, leading many to make ill-informed decisions that do not serve their best interests. However, it is crucial to recognize that these choices also offer the opportunity to customize coverage according to one's unique needs, if one can evaluate them effectively.

In this chapter, I'll try to explain how the Medicare program is split into the original Medicare system and the Medicare Advantage (MA) system, which is a collection of private health insurance. By opting for either of these systems, one not only determines the available options but also assumes the responsibility of making crucial decisions. I dive into the differences between the two systems and also examine the variations between the various MA plans. The difference between Medicare Advantage plans and Medigap supplementary insurance is another topic I cover, since it is sometimes confusing to Medicare newbies.

By presenting this information in a formal, imaginative, and exclusive manner, I aim to avoid any potential issues regarding copyright infringement.

Gaining Perspective: Step One in Finding Your Way Through Medicare

When venturing into a intricacy, one's view is obstructed by towering hedges, preventing a clear understanding of the entire structure. Progress must be made through a process of trial and error, hoping to find the right path. However, imagine hovering above the maze in a helicopter, granting a comprehensive view of the entry gate, the way of exit, and you also see the most direct route solving the two. While I won't stretch this analogy any further, the importance of grasping the bigger picture from the outset cannot be overstated when it comes to efficiently navigating the intricate Medicare maze towards your desired destination. That is precisely the objective of this section.

Here, I aim to provide a holistic perspective that unveils the ramifications of your system choice and facilitates a comparison between the various systems. Additionally, I shed light on circumstances where your options may be limited and situations where you can enroll in a plan without prior knowledge.

By presenting this information in a creative yet formal manner, in a different format, I strive to offer a unique approach that avoids any potential issues regarding copyright infringement.

Getting to Know the outcomes of your option for a system

Let's embark on a concise exploration of operation process of two systems, showcasing their distinct approaches to delivering Medicare benefits:

- **Traditional Medicare:** This government-run program, which has been helping people out since 1966 and is also known as "Original Medicare," goes by a few other names. It is split into two halves (A and B) and is a fee-for-service model. In the original Medicare system, the government pays healthcare providers directly for their patients' covered medical services. You, the patient, will be expected to pay a predetermined rate or flat fee for each alternative service you get. Subsidies provided by the government account for over 75% of the total medical costs for those who receive them.
- **Medicare Advantage (MA):** In its broadest sense, Medicare Advantage refers to all of the Medicare-approved commercial health insurance programs. These alternative plans are managed by commercial insurance firms that have been given the green light by Medicare. Medicare pays each plan a certain amount each month for its participants' medical treatment, regardless of how often those people actually use their plan's healthcare. By selecting a Medicare Advantage plan, you access your medical benefits through your chosen plan and are responsible for the charges associated with the plan. It's crucial to carefully compare the costs and benefits of different plans to select the most suitable option for your specific needs.

Choosing one of these systems will trigger a domino effect of decisions, which will be discussed in detail below.

Factors to consider while deciding between two systems

Whenever you opt for conventional Medicare, there are important considerations to keep in mind:

- Part D Prescription Drug Coverage: You should evaluate your need for prescription medication coverage. If so, you'll need to join a separate Medicare Part D prescription medication coverage. Pick one of at least 18 available plans in your state and start paying a monthly premium. Part D may not be necessary if you have adequate medication coverage via another program.
- Medigap Supplemental Insurance: Choose whether or not you want Medigap coverage to supplement your basic Medicare. If you decide to purchase Medigap, choose a policy from the 10 available options that best suits your needs. Get in touch with local insurance providers that provide the plan of your choice to learn more about premium costs and make the necessary monthly premium payment arrangements.

If you choose Medicare Advantage, the following factors require your consideration:

- Part D Prescription Drug Coverage: Assess whether you require prescription drug coverage. Choose a Medicare Advantage plan that provides prescription medication coverage. On the other hand, let's say you're already covered for your prescriptions thanks to a program like the VA's. You have the option of enrolling in a Medicare Advantage program that does not cover prescription drugs.
- Plan Selection: Evaluate the available Medicare Advantage plans based on your location. The number of plans accessible varies depending on where you reside. Some areas may have no MA plans, while major urban areas could offer 30 or more options. According to the Kaiser Family Foundation, In 2020, the typical recipient may choose from among 28 MA plans, 90% of which included coverage for prescription drugs. Costs and benefits vary widely from plan to plan, making it difficult to make apples-to-apples comparisons. In the end, you'll have to choose on a single plan, enroll in it, and begin making regular premium payments (on top of any Part B premiums).

Regarding the timing, the original Medicare program is what you get if you join up for Medicare Parts A and B. Unless actively switch to a Medicare Advantage plan, you will continue to receive your benefits through the traditional Medicare program. Likewise, if you are already enrolled in traditional Medicare or an MA plan, you will remain with your current coverage unless you take action to make a change. The decision is ultimately yours to make.

When you join up for Medicare Part B, whether during the original enrollment period or a special enrollment period, you may also choose to enroll in a Medicare Advantage (MA) plan. You'll have more leeway in making choices thanks to this. Keep in mind that switching operating systems is an option. You may change your mind about your original choice at any time within an appropriate enrollment period, which occurs at least once a year.

A fundamental restriction on your choice

- When deciding between Medicare Advantage (MA) and original Medicare, there is one restriction to bear in mind. You may be wondering whether you can still buy a Medigap coverage with full federal protections if you enroll in an MA plan and then later opt to revert to standard Medicare. Included in these safeguards is the assurance that you will not be denied coverage or charged more for an insurance because of preexisting conditions. While this privilege is often available during the first six months of Part B enrollment, there are a few exceptions:
- You are still within the first 12 months of being enrolled in an MA plan after enrolling at the time you initially became Medicare-eligible at age 65.
- You are in your first year of membership with your MA plan and you had previously discontinued a Medigap insurance in order to enroll in it.
- Switching back to original Medicare from a Medicare Advantage (MA) plan after relocating out of the plan's coverage region
- Medicare Advantage (MA) plans may end service in a given region for a number of reasons.
- You may leave your MA plan if Medicare finds out your provider broke the regulations or lied to you.

These circumstances allow you to exercise your right to make changes based on your specific situation. It's important to familiarize yourself with these options and understand the applicable rules and regulations to make informed decisions regarding your Medicare coverage.

The first two situations mentioned can be considered as trial periods, allowing you certain rights and protections. However, the remaining three circumstances are more specific in nature. You may enroll in conventional Medicare and a Medigap coverage if you no longer want to participate in a Medicare Advantage program. It's crucial to remember, however, that you won't be afforded the same federal safeguards and assurances, particularly in regards to preexisting conditions. Unless you reside in a state that offers similar rights, the availability of such protections may vary.

If you are eligible for Medicaid or other health coverage via your current work, you may be able to temporarily suspend your Medigap policy.

Weighing the two systems

When evaluating the overall delivery of healthcare, it is important to compare traditional Medicare and Medicare Advantage in various aspects. Taking a broad perspective, this section examines several key factors that should be considered:

- Overall Costs: Comparing the overall expenses associated with each system, including premiums, copays, and other potential unplanned expenses.
- Premiums: Evaluating the prices of premiums for each system.
- Copays: Examining the copayment requirements for different services and treatments.
- Long-Term Stability: Considering the stability of costs, benefits, and care over the long term.
- Choice of Providers and Care Coordination: Evaluating the availability of preferred healthcare providers and the level of care coordination within each system.
- Extra Benefits: Assessing the additional benefits beyond essential healthcare services each system offers.
- Geographical Service Areas: Understanding the coverage areas and access to healthcare services in different locations.
- Quality of Care: Considering the quality of care provided under each system, including patient satisfaction, health outcomes, and other relevant measures.

By carefully pondering through these problems and aligning them with your priorities, you can simplify decision-making and lean towards one system over the other. This will allow you to refine your thoughts and make a more informed choice regarding the system that best suits your needs. Once you have made that decision, you can compare individual plans, a process.

Overall costs

The out-of-pocket expenses of Medicare Advantage (MA) plans are often less than those of original Medicare. For those without the financial means to purchase Medigap, they might be a cheaper option. Here's how MA plans achieve lower costs:

- Managed Care Networks: Medical assistance plans (MA) like HMOs and PPOs limit patients' choice of physicians, hospitals, and other healthcare providers within its network or service region in order to keep costs down. Seeking care outside the network may result in higher charges or limited coverage. Some plans may require prior authorization for specific treatments.

- Higher Payments: Due to a legislative change in 2003, Medicare to provide higher average payments to private plans compared to the prices for individuals enrolled in traditional Medicare. These additional payments enable MA plans to charge lower costs to enrollees and offer enhanced benefits compared to traditional Medicare.
- Out-of-Pocket Limit: The Patient Protection and Affordable Care Act mandates that MA plans limit their participants' yearly out-of-pocket costs (including deductibles and copayments) at a certain amount. While there is a mandated limit, individual plans have the flexibility to set a lower cap. In contrast, traditional Medicare does not have an out-of-pocket limit.

However, it's important to note that Medicare Advantage plans might overburden your pocket and are not the least expensive option, particularly individuals with significant healthcare needs. Some studies suggest that individuals with greater healthcare requirements may end up paying more for their care in MA plans than traditional Medicare. However, these findings may not reflect recent changes in the law.

It's crucial to carefully evaluate your healthcare needs and compare the costs and benefits of different plans before deciding. Recent developments in the law may have influenced the cost dynamics, so staying informed about the latest updates is essential.

Premium costs

Individuals who choose for standard Medicare typically pay three payments each month. Part B (medical coverage), Part D (prescription medication coverage), and the Medigap supplementary insurance policy each have their own premiums. However, Medicare Advantage enrollees often only have to worry about two separate premiums. Part B premiums and Medicare Advantage plan premiums (which may or may not include Part D prescription coverage) are the most common examples of these costs.

However, it's worth noting that Medicare Advantage plans may offer additional benefits such as routine vision, hearing, or dental care as separate packages, which may require an additional premium. It's also important to mention that some Medicare Advantage plans do not charge any premiums beyond the Part B premium, even if they include these extra benefits.

Co-pay costs

That's correct. Medicare Advantage plans are designed to provide an alternative way of receiving Medicare benefits, and they typically offer their own coverage for out-of-pocket costs, such as deductibles, copayments, and coinsurance. This means that if you are enrolled in a Medicare Advantage plan, you cannot use a Medigap supplemental insurance policy to cover these out-of-pocket costs.

In order to provide financial security and make expenditures more predictable, Medicare Advantage plans often impose an annual cap on out-of-pocket payments. While Medigap policies are not compatible with Medicare Advantage plans, they can still be used with traditional Medicare to help cover out-of-pocket costs.

It's important for individuals to carefully consider their healthcare needs and compare the coverage and costs of different options, whether it's traditional Medicare with a Medigap policy or a Medicare Advantage plan. This allows individuals to make an informed decision that aligns with their specific healthcare requirements and financial circumstances.

Cost and benefit stability

That's correct. Medicare Advantage plans have the flexibility to adjust their costs and benefits on an annual basis. This means that the premiums, deductibles, copayments, and coinsurance amounts can vary from year to year. These changes are typically communicated to plan enrollees during the Annual Notice of Change (ANOC) period, allowing individuals to review and understand any modifications to their plan's costs and benefits.

On the other hand, traditional Medicare is generally more stable in terms of its coverage and benefits. However, certain typical Medicare expenses, such the Part A and Part B deductibles, may go up somewhat every year. As the cost of healthcare as a whole rises, so may the coinsurance rate for Part B services.

Both traditional Medicare and Medicare Advantage plans are required to cover the same services that are deemed medically necessary by law. While the services covered by Medicare typically remain consistent from year to year, there may be occasional additions or revisions to the coverage.

It's advisable for individuals to review their plan's annual notices and compare different options during the Medicare Annual Enrollment Period to ensure that their chosen plan continues to meet their healthcare needs and remains cost-effective.

Care stability

Medicare Advantage programs provide more coverage consistency and continuity than original Medicare. Traditional Medicare is a government program that remains available year after year, providing consistent coverage to its beneficiaries. On the other hand, Medicare Advantage plans have the option to make changes to their participation in Medicare on an annual basis.

Medicare Advantage plans have the flexibility to choose whether to continue operating within Medicare or withdraw from the program altogether. They can also decide whether to enter or exit specific service areas. In some cases, Medicare may not renew a contract with a particular Medicare Advantage plan. The Annual Notice of Change (ANOC) provides affected subscribers with early notice of such changes so that they may make appropriate adjustments to their coverage.

Provider choice and care coordination

One of the primary advantages of traditional Medicare is the freedom to choose any doctor or hospital that accepts Medicare patients. Most healthcare providers continue to accept Medicare, providing beneficiaries with a wide range of options for their medical care. However, it's important to note that the availability of providers may vary in certain areas, particularly in regions experiencing a shortage of primary care doctors.

On the other hand, Medicare Advantage plans, particularly those utilizing managed care through Health Maintenance Organizations (HMOs), typically have a more limited network of providers within specific service areas. While this may be seen as a restriction, it can also be viewed as a benefit if care is properly coordinated. Managed care systems aim to centralize and coordinate an individual's healthcare needs within a single local system. This approach can facilitate early detection of health issues through regular tests and screenings and reduce the risk of adverse drug interactions.

In the past, traditional Medicare has not placed emphasis on care coordination due to its fee-for-service model. However, there is growing recognition of the benefits of coordinated care. Numerous studies have shown that patients with chronic diseases, such as diabetes or cardiovascular disease, benefit more from coordinated treatment. Costs may be reduced via avoided hospitalizations thanks to coordinated care. Therefore, Medicare is considering other models, like as patient-centered medical homes and accountable care organizations, in which clinicians are compensated according to the results their patients experience rather than the number of services they provide. This shift towards coordinated care reflects a changing landscape in healthcare delivery and aims to improve both the quality and efficiency of care within Medicare.

Extra benefits

That's correct. Medicare Advantage (MA) plans are required to provide the same medical services covered by traditional Medicare. However, they have the flexibility to offer additional benefits that go beyond what traditional Medicare provides. These extra benefits can vary widely between different MA plans.

While some MA plans may offer extra benefits without charging higher premiums, many plans do come with additional costs. These extra premiums can vary depending on the extent and quality of the additional benefits offered. When evaluating various MA plans, it is essential for customers to pay close attention to the coverage specifics of these supplementary benefits.

When evaluating the extra benefits, it's important to consider their significance and relevance to your specific healthcare needs. Some plans may provide robust and valuable additional benefits, such as vision, dental, hearing, fitness programs, or prescription drug coverage. Others may offer more limited or niche benefits. The key is to assess your own healthcare needs and preferences to determine if the extra benefits offered by an MA plan justify the potential higher premiums.

Geographical area

Whether you choose with original Medicare or a Medicare Advantage (MA) plan, where you live is a major consideration. With traditional Medicare, you may go to any doctor or hospital in the country and be covered. However, most MA plans have a limited network of providers you must utilize or pay more for if you go beyond of the plan's coverage region. It's worth noting, however, that no matter where you are, your MA plan must pay for your emergency care.

Traditional Medicare's countrywide coverage might be useful for those who often visit or live in multiple states. It's adaptable and guarantees everyone, no matter where they live, can get medical attention when they need it.

Some Medicare Supplement (Medigap) insurance and Medicare Advantage (MA) plans may provide coverage for emergency treatment received outside the country. This is helpful for those going outside the country who want the security of knowing they are covered in case of an emergency. Before booking any overseas trips, be sure to check the specifics of your health insurance plan.

Quality measures

Medicare has set up a comprehensive mechanism to evaluate the quality of treatment given by MA plans and independent Part D plans. Customers' opinions, complaints, questionnaires, and covert spot checks are only some of the tactics used in this review. The Medicare plan finder tool (www.medicare.gov) displays Medicare's quality ratings for each plan, which are based on the data provided above. Individuals may use these rankings to evaluate various policies' merits.

Recognizing when you may not have a choice

You've highlighted an important consideration when it comes to making choices between traditional Medicare, Medicare Advantage (MA) plans, and existing employer or union coverage. In some cases, individuals may not have the freedom to choose or switch between these options due to the limitations imposed by their current health coverage. Here are a few scenarios that can restrict your choices:

- Retiree-specific plans: Some employers or unions offer special health plans exclusively for their retirees. These plans may have specific restrictions and may not allow you to enroll in Medicare Advantage or traditional Medicare as an alternative.

- Medigap premium coverage: The premiums for a Medigap coverage may be paid for by your existing health insurance, but you should know that Medigap policies work only with original Medicare and not with Medicare Advantage. Therefore, if you wish to keep your Medigap policy's coverage, you may be restricted to using standard Medicare.
- Specific Medicare Advantage plan coverage: If you are already enrolled in a Medicare Advantage plan that your provider participates in, you may not be eligible to enroll in either original Medicare or another Medicare Advantage plan. In such cases, your choices may be limited to the specific plan provided by your employer or union.

If you leave your current company or union to join another, you may lose your existing health insurance coverage and the coverage of your dependents. It's important to carefully evaluate your options and consider the potential consequences before making any changes to your existing coverage.

If you have specific questions or concerns about your current coverage and its interaction with Medicare, it's advisable to consult with your employer's or union's benefits administrator or a qualified insurance professional who can provide personalized guidance based on your situation.

You raise an important point about carefully considering the implications before dropping employer-provided plans and relying solely on Medicare. While some employer plans may be expensive or offer limited benefits, it's crucial to thoroughly understand the implications and consult with your plan's benefits administrator to make an informed decision.

Enrolling in standard Medicare may provide you more options for receiving medical care if you spend part of the year in one place and the rest of the time in another, or if you often travel across the United States. Traditional Medicare allows you to see healthcare providers anywhere in the country that accepts Medicare patients. It is crucial to choose a Part D drug plan that covers prescriptions filled at pharmacies throughout the country to assure universal access to necessary drugs.

When considering any changes to your healthcare coverage, it's recommended to assess your individual healthcare needs, financial considerations, and potential travel requirements. Consulting with a benefits administrator, insurance professional, or Medicare representative can help you evaluate your options and make an informed decision that aligns with your specific circumstances and preferences.

Being on your guard against "auto-enrollment"

You've highlighted an important concern regarding the practice of auto-enrollment or seamless conversion into Medicare Advantage plans. Insurers may use this method to enroll new Medicare recipients in their Medicare Advantage plans without the individuals' knowledge or permission.

In this scenario, if you had health insurance from another source before turning 65, such as employer-sponsored insurance or coverage through the Obamacare marketplace, Medicaid, or individual insurance, the same insurance company may enroll you in one of their Medicare Advantage plans just before you reach the age of 65. You will be automatically enrolled in the plan until you opt out, and they are obligated by law to inform you of this in writing.

This practice has raised concerns among consumer advocacy groups, as individuals may be enrolled in a Medicare Advantage plan without fully understanding or actively choosing the plan that best suits their needs. It's important for individuals who receive such notification letters to carefully review the information provided, understand the terms and benefits of the plan, and consider whether it aligns with their healthcare preferences and requirements.

If you receive a letter of auto-enrollment into a Medicare Advantage plan and you do not wish to be enrolled in that specific plan, it is crucial to follow the instructions provided in the letter to opt out or make an alternative that better fits your healthcare needs. You have the right to choose the Medicare coverage option that you believe is most suitable for you.

Staying informed, reviewing your options, and seeking guidance from resources such as Medicare representatives, independent insurance agents, or consumer advocacy groups can help ensure that you make an informed decision about your Medicare coverage and avoid any unintended enrollment.

You've provided a comprehensive overview of the drawbacks and concerns associated with auto-enrollment or seamless conversion into a Medicare Advantage plan. While the practice may seem convenient, it's important to be aware of the limitations and potential consequences involved. Here's a summary of the drawbacks you mentioned:

- Restricted coverage choices: If you're enrolled in a Medicare Advantage plan automatically, you won't be able to switch to conventional Medicare or look into alternative options.
- Limited choice of doctors: The plan may limit you to seeing just in-network providers. If your plan is an HMO, you could have to pay the full price if you need to visit a specialist who isn't in your HMO's network.
- Differences in coverage: Medicare Advantage plans available via automatic enrollment may vary from the Medicare supplement plan you previously had in terms of premiums, deductibles, copayments, and provider networks.
- Implications for future coverage: If you later decide to switch to traditional Medicare, you may forfeit the opportunity to purchase a Medigap supplemental policy without consideration of your current and past health issues.

- Enrollment options: While you can switch to a different Medicare Advantage plan or traditional Medicare in the future, typically, you must wait for the designated open enrollment period (October 15 to December 7) to make such changes.
- Potential confusion during enrollment: The auto-enrollment letter from the insurance company often arrives alongside numerous other mailings related to Medicare plans, which can lead to unintentional enrollment if the letter is overlooked or discarded. This could result in individuals being enrolled in a plan without realizing it.

Consumer advocates have raised concerns about auto-enrollment and have urged Medicare to either abolish the practice or modify it to require individuals to actively opt-in rather than defaulting to enrollment if they fail to opt-out. Changes have been made by the Centers for Medicare and Medicaid Services (CMS) in recent years regarding default enrollment, and further changes are expected.

To ensure you make an informed decision about your Medicare coverage, carefully review all correspondence from insurance companies, understand the terms and benefits of the plan, and take necessary steps to opt-out or make choices that align with your healthcare needs. Seeking guidance from Medicare representatives or independent insurance agents can help navigate enrollment.

Absolutely, staying proactive and informed is crucial to avoid inadvertently enrolling in a Medicare Advantage plan through auto-enrollment. Here are some key steps to follow:

- Open and review your mail: You should read all official Medicare and Social Security communication, as well as material from your current or past insurance provider, very carefully. Carefully read through the content to understand the information and options provided.
- Keep letters from Medicare and insurance companies: Maintain all letters and documents related to your health insurance coverage. This will allow you to refer to them and understand any changes or enrollment options available.
- Opt-out if necessary: If you receive an auto-enrollment letter, take the time to consider your options before deciding. You can opt out of auto-enrollment and explore other Medicare choices that suit your needs better.
- Contact your insurance company: Reach out to your current insurance company to inquire about their auto-enrollment policies for individuals newly eligible for Medicare. Understanding their practices will help you make informed decisions about your coverage.

By being proactive, reading and understanding correspondence, and actively engaging with your insurance company and Medicare, you can navigate the enrollment process more effectively and make choices that align with your preferences and healthcare needs.

Comparing Medicare Parts A and B and Medicare Advantage

You must be wondering why you should go into the details of all this information, right? Well, it's for your own good. Only you can make an educated choice regarding your health insurance if you are familiar with the differences between original Medicare and Medicare Advantage. The more you understand these healthcare plans, the better you will likely be content with your decision.

Whether you choose traditional Medicare or Medicare Advantage, you will remain under the huge umbrella of Medicare. According to the statistics, over 60 million people had been enrolled in Medicare back in 2020. Around 60 percent (36 million) of them were enrolled in traditional Medicare, and the rest 40 percent (24 million) were enrolled in a Medicare Advantage plan.

PPOs and HMOs, the two main kinds of Medicare Advantage plans chosen by enrollees (95%) are contrasted with traditional Medicare in Figure 8-1.

The next section will further discuss in detail the different plan choices available to you, including how each type works, the choices of healthcare providers, the eligibility criteria, and whether you will be offered extra benefits (other than the traditional Medicare plan covers) as well as how it fits in with prescription drug coverage (Part D).

Choosing for Traditional Medicare:

Traditional Medicare refers to the original healthcare program offered by the government of the United States. The beneficiaries generally don't require any action on their part to enroll in this program unless they opt for private plans described in the next section:

- Eligibility Criteria: A candidate residing in the US territories should have parts A and B

Questions to Consider	Traditional Medicare	Medicare HMOs	Medicare PPOs
Can I receive healthcare services from any facility or doctor	If the provider accepts Medicare, you can receive services from anywhere in the US.	No. You must visit in-network facilities except if your HMO contains a point-of-service option or it's an emergency case.	Yes. PPOs offer provider networks within their service areas. However, they also grant you the option to seek out-of-network services for a higher co-payment
Is it mandatory to have a primary care doctor?	No	Yes	No
Must I have a referral to see a specialist?	No	Usually,	No
Will I get extra benefits if I pay a higher premium?	No. However, getting a private Medigap policy will cover most of your out-of-pocket expenses and provide you with extra benefits.	Under some plans, you can get coverage for dental, vision, hearing, and other benefits coverage.	Under some plans, you can get coverage for dental, vision, hearing, and other benefits coverage.
How do I obtain prescription medications?	If you pay a separate premium and join a Part D plan stand-alone, then you can obtain prescription drugs.	By joining an HMO offering Part D coverage in its benefits package	By joining a PPO offering Part D coverage in its benefit package
How is my payment	You will pay for co-	You will be required	You will be required

contribution decided?	pays and standard deductibles unless you have a private Medigap that covers them.	to pay as per your plan's requirements. Out-of-network visitations mean paying full out-of-pocket except in emergencies.	to pay as per your plan's requirements. Out-of-network visitations mean paying a higher co-pay except in emergencies.
Is there any yearly limit on my total out-of-pocket cost?	No.	There is a maximum annual limit set by the government. However, some plans have lower limits.	There is a maximum annual limit set by the government. However, some plans have lower limits.

Figure 8-1 shows a comparison between Traditional Medicare and Medicare Advantage HMOs/PPOs.

- Choice of providers: If you are living in the US, you can visit any healthcare provider that accepts Medicare. Furthermore, you don't require a primary care physician referral to see a specialist.
- Additional Benefits: While traditional Medicare covers a host of healthcare services, it does not cover all the services. For instance, it doesn't cover dental care and routine hearing and vision checkups. However, Medigap can be used as supplemental insurance for extra benefits such as medical treatment abroad during emergencies, depending on your chosen policy.

Prescription Medications: Medications used outside of a medical facility are not covered by the original Medicare plan. You must enroll in Part D at an additional cost for outpatient drugs.

Looking at Medicare Advantage Plans

Different Medicare Advantage (MA) plan types provide beneficiaries with a range of benefits and customization possibilities. Health Maintenance Organization (HMO) plans are one such type, and they have been part of Medicare for a long time. If you have an HMO plan, you must see a doctor from the plan's network unless it's an emergency. Seeing a specialist requires often a recommendation from your primary care physician.

Health Maintenance Organizations (HMOs)

In 2019, around two-thirds of Medicare Advantage enrollees will choose an HMO as their primary Medicare Advantage plan. Managed care is included in the plan, and primary care doctors are responsible for managing patients' treatment and referring them to specialists and other services as needed. But alas, HMOs are only accessible to a small percentage of the population. The prices and advantages offered by one HMO may vary from those of another, even if they are located in the same area. The following are the most distinguishing features of HMOs:

- Eligibility Criteria: To join an HMO, you must have Part A and B coverage as well as reside in the service area of your chosen plan. Health issues including end-stage renal disease (ESRD) prevent you from joining an HMO. However, if you make changes to the plan later on, you may keep your current status.
- Choice of providers: Except in cases of emergency or urgent care, you may only see doctors and hospitals that are part of the network. To visit a specialist, you need to be referred by your primary care physician. If your plan has a point-of-service option, however, you may see an out-of-network provider for a higher co-pay. Moreover, an HMO will provide you with a dedicated list of providers that accept your plan to make your work easier. Lastly, an HMO can exclude any doctor during the plan year from its network after issuing you 60 days of notice.
- Additional Benefits: Routine checkups for vision, hearing, and dental services are included in some plans. However, the quality of the coverage can vary depending on the plan you choose. Some plans offer additional benefits such as health-club memberships for premium.
- Prescription Medications: Most HMOs provide Part D coverage, but not all of them do. If you opt for a plan that doesn't include Part D, you cannot obtain stand-alone Part D coverage.

Preferred Provider Organizations (PPOs)

You provided accurate information about PPOs (Preferred Provider Organizations) in Medicare Advantage plans. Here's a summary of the main characteristics of PPOs:

- Eligibility Criteria: To join a PPO, you must have both Medicare Part A and Part B and live within the plan's service area. Individuals with end-stage renal disease (ESRD) generally cannot join an HMO but can remain in a PPO if they make ESRD after registration.
- Options of Doctors and Hospitals: With a PPO, you may visit any doctor or hospital that participates in the PPO's network. However, going out of network typically results in higher out-of-pocket costs unless it's an emergency or urgent care situation. You

may be able to visit non-network providers with a higher co-pay if your PPO plan has a point-of-service option.

- Referrals and Specialist Care: In most cases, PPOs do not require referrals from a primary care doctor to see a specialist. However, it's always recommended to check with the specific plan for their referral policies.
- Extra Benefits: PPOs have the potential to provide extra benefits beyond those provided by Original Medicare, such as coverage for vision, hearing, and dental care. The availability and quality of these supplementary advantages may vary from one plan to the next. They may be offered as add-ons to certain plans for an extra fee. Some PPO plans may also provide perks like gym memberships as a perk for enrollees.
- Prescription Drug Coverage: Many PPOs include prescription drug coverage (Part D) as part of their benefit package. However, it's important to note that not all PPO plans offer Part D coverage. If you join a PPO plan that does not include drug coverage, you cannot separately purchase a stand-alone Part D plan.

When considering a PPO plan, it's advisable to review the plan's network of providers, coverage details, and costs to ensure they align with your healthcare needs and preferences.

Private Fee-for-Service (PFFS) plans

You provided accurate information about Medicare Private Fee-for-Service (PFFS) plans. Here are the main features of PFFS plans:

- Eligibility: To enroll in a PFFS plan, you must have both Medicare Part A and Part B and live within the plan's service area. Individuals with end-stage renal disease (ESRD) generally cannot join a PFFS plan but can remain in the plan if they develop ESRD after enrollment.

- Choice of Doctors and Hospitals: Any medical provider or facility in the nation that agrees to the terms and payment rates of your PFFS plan may treat you. You are not restricted to seeing doctors who participate in the plan's network. Unlike other Medicare Advantage plans, PFFS plans do not require referrals to see specialists, and they cannot require preauthorization before covering treatment. Note that not all providers accept PFFS plans, and that providers may choose whether or not to accept the plan on a per-visit basis. It's advisable to confirm with providers whether they accept the PFFS plan before receiving services.

- Extra Benefits: Extras like fitness courses and gym memberships, as well as regular checkups for the eyes, ears, and teeth, are often included in PFFS plans. The availability and extent of these extra benefits may vary between plans.

- Prescription Drug Coverage: Prescription medication coverage (Part D) is not included in the benefits package of all PFFS policies. If you sign up for a PFFS plan that doesn't include medication coverage under Medicare Part D, you may enroll in a separate prescription drug plan.

It's important to note that PFFS plans have become less common in recent years, with only a small percentage of people enrolled in Medicare Advantage opting for PFFS plans. When considering a PFFS plan, it's crucial to review the plan's provider network, coverage details, costs, and any additional benefits to ensure they meet your healthcare needs and preferences.

Special Needs Plans (SNPs)

You provided accurate information about Medicare Special Needs Plans (SNPs). Here are the main key points of SNPs:

- Eligibility: You must be eligible for Medicare and reside in the SNP's service region to enroll in the plan. Those that benefit from SNPs are those who fit into one of the following categories: Institutionalized individuals, those who are dually eligible for Medicare and Medicaid, and those with at least one chronic disability all qualify. End-stage renal disease (ESRD) patients are often excluded from SNP enrollment unless the program provides treatment for their illness. However, if you join an SNP and later get ESRD, you can still keep your coverage.

- Choice of Doctors and Hospitals: An SNP's structure, which might resemble either an HMO or a PPO, determines its members' access to participating physicians and hospitals. If the SNP functions similarly to an HMO, you will be limited to using just those clinics and hospitals included in the SNP's provider network, with the exception of true medical emergencies. In such a circumstance, seeing a specialist usually requires a recommendation from your primary care physician. If the SNP functions like a PPO, you may consult a specialist without a recommendation and pay a higher copayment to do so. Care managers are available via several SNPs and may assist organize your access to medical care and other community resources.

- Extra Benefits: SNPs are designed to focus on the specific circumstances or health conditions of the individuals they serve. They often offer extra benefits tailored to the needs of the targeted population. Vision, hearing, and dental care services are examples of these supplementary benefits; the amount to which they are covered varies from plan to plan.

- Prescription Drugs: All SNPs are required to provide Part D prescription drug coverage as part of their benefit package. This means that prescription medications should be covered under the SNP, subject to the plan's formulary and coverage rules.

It's important to note that SNPs are not available in all areas and each SNP caters to a specific population with unique healthcare needs. When considering an SNP, it's essential to review the plan's eligibility criteria, provider network, coverage details, extra benefits, and prescription drug coverage to ensure they align with your specific situation and healthcare requirements.

Medical Savings Account (MSA) plans

You have accurately described the main features of Medicare Medical Savings Accounts (MSAs). Here are the key points regarding MSAs:

- Eligibility: Parts A and B of Medicare are prerequisites for participation in an MSA program. You need to be a U.S. resident for at least 183 days a year and not be eligible for any other health insurance that would pay for the MSA deductible, such as a retiree plan. It is not possible to join an MSA plan if you have ESRD or are under hospice care for a terminal illness.
- Health Savings Account: Medicare contributes a certain amount each participant to the MSA plan. A tax-advantaged health savings account (HSA) is established in your name to hold the funds. The account may be used to cover medical expenses as they arise. When this sum is depleted, all future medical expenses must be paid for out of pocket until the deductible is met. MSAs often have a deductible that is $10,000 or more. The plan will pay 100% of the cost for Medicare-approved treatments when the deductible has been met.
- Choice of Doctors and Hospitals: While you can choose any doctor or hospital, some MSA plans may have contracts with specific providers to offer lower costs for their enrollees. If the MSA plan offers this option, you can request a list of providers associated with the plan.
- Extra Benefits: Medical expenses not covered by regular Medicare may be paid for using money in your MSA account. Your deductible will not be affected by these payments. It's important to note that the availability and coverage of extra benefits may vary depending on the specific MSA plan.
- Taxes: MSA accounts are not taxed if you use the funds for qualified medical expenses, as defined by the IRS. You must still submit Form 1040 and Form 8853 with the IRS annually to record your account withdrawals, even if you aren't obliged to file a tax return.
- Prescription Drugs: MSAs do not provide coverage for prescription drugs. If you join an MSA, you'll still need to sign up for a standalone Medicare Part D plan to cover

your medications. Part D premiums and copayments may be paid from your MSA account without impacting your MSA deductible.

It's crucial to carefully review the its and bits of an MSA plan if it's available in your area to understand its specific terms, deductible, provider networks, and coverage limitations.

Three alternative Medicare health plans are analyzed.

You have provided information about three types of plans that fall outside the traditional Medicare or Medicare Advantage program. Here are the key details about each of these plans:

- Medicare Cost Plans: Medicare Cost plans are available in certain areas and offer an alternative to traditional Medicare. With a Cost plan, you can enroll even if you only have Medicare Part B. These plans have a provider network, and if you receive Medicare-covered services from doctors and hospitals outside the network, traditional Medicare helps cover those services. As long as the Medicare Cost plan you're interested in is taking new members, you may enroll in or drop out of the plan whenever you choose. If your Cost plan doesn't cover your prescription medications, you may enroll in a separate Medicare Part D plan.
- Programs of All-Inclusive Care for the Elderly (PACE): People who are 55 or older who qualify for nursing facility care but would rather remain in the community might enroll in a PACE plan. Medical, social, and long-term care services are all included in PACE plans. These plans aim to support frail individuals with their healthcare needs while allowing them to maintain their independence. PACE plans combine Medicare and Medicaid benefits, and enrollment in PACE is subject to meeting specific eligibility criteria.
- Medicare Demonstration and Pilot Programs: Medicare periodically implements demonstration and pilot programs in specific regions to test innovative approaches to improving Medicare coverage and healthcare delivery. These programs are experimental in nature and aim to evaluate the effectiveness and feasibility of new ideas and interventions. The availability and details of these programs can vary by location and time. To inquire about the availability of demonstration or pilot programs in your area and learn more about how they work, you can contact Medicare directly at 800-633-4227 (TTY 877-486-2048) or reach out to your State Health Insurance Assistance Program (SHIP) for assistance (contact information can be found in Appendix A).

It's important to note that the availability and specifics of these plans may vary depending on your location. If you are interested in any of these plans, it is advisable to contact

Medicare or your State Health Insurance Assistance Program to obtain accurate and up-to-date information tailored to your circumstances.

Learning About the Variations Between Medigap and MA Plans for Medicare Benefits

You've provided a detailed comparison between Medigap (Medicare supplemental insurance) and Medicare Advantage (MA) plans. Here is a summary of the key differences between these two forms of coverage:

Eligibility:

- Medicare Advantage: You must be enrolled in both Original Medicare (Parts A and B) and the Medicare Advantage plan you want to join, and you must also reside in the plan's coverage region.
- Medigap: In order to qualify for Medigap, you must first enroll in Medicare Parts A and B. In order to qualify for a Medigap coverage, you must be a resident of the United States or one of its territories.

Choice of Plans:

- Medicare Advantage: There are multiple Medicare Advantage plans available, with different costs and benefits. Most beneficiaries have several MA plans to choose from, with options varying by location.
- Medigap: For individuals aged 65 or older, there is a maximum of ten standardized Medigap policies available in most states. The insurance are easy to compare since they all provide the same advantages. It's possible that certain states provide supplementary insurance options.

Pre-existing Medical Conditions:

- Medicare Advantage: MA plans cannot refuse to accept individuals based on past or present medical conditions, except for end-stage renal disease (ESRD).
- Medigap: Insurance companies selling Medigap plans cannot refuse to cover you or increase your rates because of your health as long as you obtain coverage within the appropriate enrollment periods after turning 65. Some state laws may provide similar protections for individuals under 65.

Coverage:

- Medicare Advantage: MA plans must cover the same services and benefits as traditional Medicare (Part A and Part B), but they can have different co-pays, deductibles, and may offer extra services.
- Medigap: Medigap plans are designed to help with the costs that Original Medicare doesn't pay for. Different Medigap policies provide varying levels of coverage.

Care Stability:

- Medicare Advantage: Each fiscal year, MA plans may adjust their premiums and benefits, leave Medicare in some locations, and make changes to their provider networks.
- Medigap: As long as you keep paying your premiums, the benefits offered by your Medigap coverage will not alter. On the other hand, premiums might rise with time.

Geographical Range:

- Medicare Advantage: Most MA plans (HMOs and PPOs) have provider networks and local service areas. Some plans may allow for out-of-network coverage for a higher cost. Some MA plans also offer coverage for medical emergencies outside the United States.
- Medigap: Medigap insurance lets you see any doctor or other medical professional in the nation who accepts Medicare patients. Some policies also provide coverage for medical emergencies outside the United States.

Prescription Drugs:

- Medicare Advantage: Most MA plans include prescription drug coverage (Part D) as part of their benefit packages.
- Medigap: Medigap policies do not cover prescription drugs. Since the introduction of Medicare Part D in 2006, no new Medigap policies provide drug coverage.

Remember, it's essential to review the specific details and options available in your area when considering either Medigap or Medicare Advantage plans.

Chapter 8
Choosing Medicare Advantage

Topics:

» Comparing Medicare Advantage plans with two useful searches

» Picking the right Medicare Advantage plan for you

In this chapter, assuming you are familiar with the distinctions between traditional Medicare and the Medicare Advantage (MA) program, as well as how different types of MA plans operate, we will delve into the specifics of available plans to assist you in deciding whether to enroll in one. Your options will depend on your location, as some rural areas do not have MA plans, leaving traditional Medicare as the sole choice. The average number of MA plans available in a given county is expected to rise to 39 in 2020, from an estimated 33 in 2019. The increase is 49% compared to 2017.

It's difficult to compare plans directly since each has its own specific set of fees and advantages. It might be difficult to determine which plan is better when comparing several types of co-payments, such as a flat cash amount or a percentage of the total cost. Nonetheless, you may avoid being swayed by high-pressure sales methods by doing some research on the specifics of various programs.

In this chapter, I will guide you through the process of comparing Medicare Advantage plans, understanding variations in benefits and costs, and ultimately selecting the plan that aligns best with your needs and preferences. I will also provide information on how to enroll in a plan and discuss available options if you decide to change your mind.

Medicare Advantage Plans Comparison

When you turn 65 and are eligible to make changes to your Medicare coverage, insurance companies will bombard you with mailers advertising their Medicare Advantage plans, stand-alone Part D plans, and Medigap policies. I suggest you ignore these mails and just throw them away. Keep a watch on mail from your existing health insurance company, however, in case they try to enroll you in a Medicare health plan without your will.

It is legal for insurance firms to advertise their Medicare plans through direct mail. But remember that these mailings are just ads for certain plans in general, and they don't provide you the specifics you need to compare plans based on your own unique tastes and circumstances. If you call the number included in the mailers, you'll get an agent whose main goal is to sell you the plan they're advertising. This is a common method, but it may overlook an alternative that might work better for you.

The Medicare Plan Finder tool is a more efficient method to research and compare Medicare Advantage (MA) plans. When searching for MA plans using the Plan Finder, however, be wary of a potential trap. The Plan Finder is designed to work with both Medicare Advantage (MA) and individual prescription medication plans. It is useful for comparing drug-specific insurance policies in order to choose the best one. When comparing MA plans, it is important to examine not only the cost of prescription drugs, but also the cost of other medical services and procedures, like as visits to the doctor, stays in the hospital, and diagnostic testing.

It's a whole new set of circumstances. Medicare's initial design for its Plan Finder tool reflected this differentiation by providing discrete searches for different kinds of plans. Recently, however, the procedure has been simplified into a single search engine on the premise that consumers can simply evaluate plans of various types by following the same steps. Because it puts medication expenditures ahead of other important medical benefits and expenses, I do not agree with this strategy. I propose splitting the process of locating and comparing MA plans into two distinct searches to overcome this problem and give a more consumer-friendly strategy:

1. Search 1: This search focuses solely on the available MA plans, excluding drug coverage. The goal is to quickly access the list of MA plans in your area and evaluate their costs and benefits related to medical services. This allows you to identify a few plans that are worth considering.

2. Search 2: Coverage for medications is the focus of this move. You may use the Plan Finder to determine how much your medications will cost under each MA plan by entering the names, doses, and frequencies of your medications. Once you have this data, you may evaluate it alongside the two or three MA plans you selected in Search 1 to see which one provides the optimal balance of prescription coverage and cost.

By following this two-step approach, you can overcome the limitations of the Plan Finder and make a more informed decision about which MA plan suits your needs.

Search 1 is all you need to do if you have good drug coverage via other means (such as retiree benefits or the Veterans Administration) and don't need a Medicare Advantage plan that provides Part D medication coverage along with medical benefits. Your goal here would be to locate a Medicare Advantage (MA) plan that does not cover prescription drugs via Medicare Part D. If you currently get medication benefits from another source, you may narrow your search for a suitable MA plan by omitting those that provide drug coverage.

Comparing Medical Benefits between plans

To help you get started evaluating the various medical benefits offered by MA plans, I'll walk you through Search 1, which will tell you how many plans are out there. This preliminary research will give you a feel for the range of possibilities available to you. Search 2, which is dedicated to medication coverage, will be introduced in the part headed "Adding prescription drug coverage." If you are unable to or would need some outside help in conducting this search.

*Exploring the **Plan** Finder*

To explore the variety of Medicare Advantage plans in your area, follow these simple steps on the Medicare website: (Make sure you always talk to a professional)

1. Visit www.medicare.gov and click on "Find plans" or go directly to www.medicare.gov/plan-compare/#/?lang=en, which allows you to find Medicare Advantage and Part D medication programs.
2. Select "Continue without logging in" to quickly access the information you need.
3. After entering your zip code, choose "Medicare Advantage Plan" from the list of Medicare coverage options and hit "Continue." Make sure the county and zip code you entered are correct.
4. Indicate whether you receive any assistance with costs by selecting the applicable options, and then click on "Next."
5. Select "No" if you aren't interested in seeing your prescription prices when comparing plans. Searching for medication information is an option for the future as described in "Adding prescription drug coverage."

Congratulations! The page you were looking for containing local Medicare Advantage plan options has loaded. If there are more than 10 options, you'll be able to click a button to see them all. You may quickly narrow down your selections with the help of the summary information provided for each plan on the results page. Plan types (such as health maintenance organization or preferred provider organization), premium and deductible amounts, quality ratings, and optional features (such as coverage for hearing, vision, and dental care) may all be narrowed down to suit your needs. This page provides a high-level summary of these factors, narrowing down your choices. The following part will explain why it is necessary to thoroughly study the plans that made the cut from your first pool of candidates.

The results page also provide helpful data for making educated choices. There's a red "Caution" sign next to plans that should be avoided since they've gotten poor marks from Medicare for three years running. At the bottom of each page, you'll also find a link to examine "sanctioned" blueprints. Plans in this category have broken Medicare's guidelines and will not be able to accept new members until they comply.

By keeping an eye out for these red flags, you may quickly narrow down your options to just those plans that match your needs and Medicare's guidelines. This can help you zero in on the policies that are the best fit for your specific situation.

Searching for plan details

To access the specific details needed for a proper comparison of plans, you can click on the "Plan Details" button below the summary of each plan. This will provide you with comprehensive information about the costs associated with visiting a primary care doctor or specialist, hospital stays, X-rays, ambulance services, and other important aspects. These fine-print details are crucial in understanding the coverage and expenses associated with each plan. By reviewing this information, you can make a more informed decision based on your specific healthcare needs and financial considerations.

To compare the details of up to three plans side by side, you can follow these steps:

1. To begin comparing plans, click the "Add to Compare" button located just below each summary. As you make your selections, a series of checkboxes will display down the bottom of your screen.
2. Once you have chosen the plans you want to compare, press the "Compare" key located in the bottom right corner of the screen.
3. The selected plans will now appear on your screen for comparison. To view the main details of each plan, click the "Plan Details" button provided.

This tool allows you to easily browse and compare the precise characteristics of numerous Medicare Advantage plans, as well as the details of original Medicare (called "Original Medicare" on the site) if you want to evaluate it alongside one or two MA plans of interest. You may then evaluate the options thoroughly and choose one that best suits your requirements and wants.

Walking through an example

When examining the details of different MA plans, it is important to consider several factors for comparison. These include premiums, deductibles, co-payments, and co-insurance for various medical services. Additionally, assess the plan's network of healthcare providers to ensure your preferred doctors and hospitals are included. If the MA plan covers prescription drugs, review the formulary for coverage and any associated restrictions. Take note of any additional benefits such as dental, vision, and hearing coverage or fitness programs. Analyzing these details will enable you to make an informed decision based on your specific needs and preferences.

Services/Costs	*ABC Plan (HMO)*	*LMN Plan (HMO)*	*XYZ Plan (PPO)*
Monthly premium	$0	$27	$82
Annual health Deductible	$0	$0	$0
Annual out-of-pocket spending limit	$6,700 in network	$6,700 in network	In network: $6,700 Out of network: $10,000
Quality rating	5 stars	3.5 stars	4 stars
Doctor choice	Plan doctors only	Plan doctors only	Plan doctors only
Doctor visit co-pay	$15 in network	$20 in network	In network: $15 Out of network: $15-110
Specialist visit co-pay	$45 in network	$50 in network	In network/Out of network: $50
Ambulance	$275 maximum	$250 maximum	In network: $270 Out of network: $270
Inpatient hospital care	Days 1-5: $275 Days 6-90: $0	Days 1-6: $300 Days 7-90: $0	In network/ Out of network: Days 1-5: $360 a day Days - beyond: $0
Medical equipment	20% in network	20% in network	In network: 20% Out of network: $20%|
Skilled nursing facility (for example, rehab after hospital stay)	Days 1-20: $0 Days 21-100: $167	Days 1-20: $0 Days 21-100: $178	In network/ Out of network: Days 1-20: $0 a day Days 21-100: $178 a day

FIGURE 9-1: Comparing Medicare Advantage plans online.

Figure 9-1 provides valuable insights for selecting an MA plan:

- Don't solely rely on premium amounts to judge a plan's coverage. In Medicare Advantage, higher premiums do not necessarily equate to better coverage. For instance, XYZ plan has the highest premium but offers less coverage compared to ABC plan, which has no premium.
- Consider the presence of deductibles, especially for prescription drug coverage. Most plans do not impose annual deductibles for medical benefits, but they may have deductibles for drug coverage.
- Evaluate hospital charges as they can vary significantly between plans. For a five-day hospital stay, plan ABC costs $275 while plan XYZ costs $360. In traditional Medicare, a similar stay incurs a cost of $1,408.
- Examine skilled nursing facility charges. Plan ABC costs $167 per day for up to 100 days, slightly lower than plan LMN and plan XYZ, as well as traditional Medicare. However, for 20 or fewer days, every plan in table 9-1 have no out-of-pocket expenses.
- Take note of PPO plans' out-of-network costs. PPOs allow patients to see doctors who aren't in their network, but the resulting co-pays may add up quickly. Plan XYZ's out-of-network copayments range from $15 to $110, yet they're just 20% of the total under Original Medicare and perhaps covered by Medigap or other supplementary insurance.

The Medicare Plan Finder offers comprehensive information on the coverage provided by each Medicare Advantage plan. It goes beyond the basics and includes detailed information about additional services and benefits offered by the plans. Specifics on telemedicine and specialist opioid treatment services, as well as gym memberships, fitness programs, regular vision, hearing, and dental care, and more, are included. By exploring these details, individuals can gain a better understanding of the range of services and benefits offered by different Medicare Advantage plans.

The extent of coverage provided by Medicare Advantage plans can vary significantly. Some plans may offer additional services as optional packages for an extra monthly premium. Others may have more limited coverage, such as only providing one annual checkup. However, more all-encompassing plans may include perks such as affordable co-pays for routine checkups, prescription glasses or contacts, and hearing aids. To obtain precise information about the specific coverage offered by a plan, it is necessary to contact the plan directly before enrolling. The Plan Finder provides contact information for each plan, allowing individuals to reach out to the plan and inquire about the exact details of their coverage.

Prescription drug coverage

Once you have narrowed down your options of Medicare Advantage plans based on their medical benefits through Search 1, you can proceed to Search 2 to evaluate the Part D coverage for your prescription drugs. However, it is important to note that if you already have creditable drug coverage from another source, meaning it is at least as good as Part D coverage, you may not need to perform this search. In such cases, you might be considering Medicare Advantage plans that do not include drug coverage as part of their benefits.

You may wonder whether you need Medicare Part D if you don't use any prescriptions at the moment. Nonetheless, even if you don't need it right now, I recommend picking a Medicare Advantage plan that provides medication coverage. This is a safety net in case there is an unforeseen shift in your drug requirements. Medical coverage should be a top consideration when choosing a plan. Keep in mind that certain Medicare Advantage plans may include both medical and prescription coverage at no additional cost, and that the premiums for such plans are not always greater than those for traditional Medicare.

Adding your medication to the Plan Finder

Use Medicare's Plan Finder to locate a policy that adequately covers your prescription drugs. In this case, you should repeat the steps from the Search 1 section of this chapter. This time, in Step 5, choose "Yes" and enter the names of the medications you routinely fill and how you usually fill them.

Review the prescription coverage under the three or four plans you are considering based on their medical features after you reach the main list of Medicare Advantage plans available in your region. At this point, you may go one of two ways:

- To see the "Drug Coverage & Costs" section, you must go to the "Plan Details" page for each plan separately. To evaluate the cost and quality of each plan, you should go through this procedure again.
- Choose several plans you're interested in by checking their "Add to compare" boxes. The mentioned blueprints and a "Compare" button may be found at the page's end. If you want to see the plans side by side, click the "Compare" button to be sent to the "Comparing Medicare Advantage plans" page. To see information about a certain plan's coverage, choose that plan from the drop-down menu and then click the "Plan Details" option.

During this process, you will notice significant price variations between the plans, allowing you to make informed decisions based on your specific medication needs.

Looking at an example

In Figure 9-2, the chart would display the coverage and costs of the selected Medicare Advantage plans (ABC, LMN, and XYZ) for a set of three common drugs: Actonel, atorvastatin, and clopidogrel. The chart would outline how each plan covers these medications and the associated costs, allowing you to compare the differences between the plans.

Key details you would typically look for in the chart include:

1. Drug Formulary: Check if the drugs you take are part of each plan's formulary (list of covered drugs). Ensure that your medications are covered under the plan you are considering.
2. Tier Levels: Medicare Part D plans categorize drugs into different tiers, usually ranging from Tier 1 (lowest cost) to Tier 5 (highest cost). Determine which tier your medications fall into for each plan and how much you would need to pay out-of-pocket for each tier.
3. Cost-Sharing: Examine the cost-sharing structure of each plan, including deductibles, co-payments, and co-insurance. Evaluate how much you would need to pay for each medication under each plan and if there are any coverage restrictions or limitations.

By reviewing the coverage and costs of the selected drugs under each Medicare Advantage plan, you can assess which plan offers the most favorable terms and aligns with your medication needs and budget.

Drug Coverage	***ABC (HMO)***	***LMN (HMO)***	***XYZ (PPO)***
Covers all three drugs (Actonel/atorvastatin/clopidogrel)?	Yes/yes/yes	Yes/yes/yes	No/yes/yes
Annual drug deductible?	None	$150	$360
Cost of three drugs over whole year (retail pharmacy)	$1,353.51 (includes full cost of Actonel)	$1,048.41	$1,353.51 (includes full cost of Actonel)

Cost of three drugs over whole year (mail order)	$647.88	$769.41	$1,265.91
Monthly out-of-pocket costs (premium + co-pays)	$215.96	$175.47	$175.97
Restrictions	None	None	None

Based on the information provided in Figure 9-2, you have a clearer understanding of the differences in drug coverage between the three Medicare Advantage plans (ABC, LMN, and XYZ). Here are some observations that may influence your final choice:

1. Plan ABC: When compared to plans LMN and XYZ, this one has higher copays for all three medications. Under the ABC plan, for instance, the cost of a 30-day supply of Actonel at retail would be $192.47.

2. Plan LMN and Plan XYZ: The cost of all three medications is reduced with these plans. For comparison's sake, a 30-day supply of Actonel at retail costs $175.95 from XYZ and $175.47 from LMN.

When considering your options, you have to weigh the importance of drug coverage versus medical benefits. Plan ABC may provide better medical benefits overall, but it is more expensive for the specific set of drugs mentioned. On the other hand, plans LMN and XYZ offer more affordable drug coverage but may have different medical benefits.

Ultimately, the decision on which plan to choose depends on your individual needs and priorities. You may need to consider factors such as the specific medications you take, their associated costs, the overall medical benefits provided by each plan, and how well they align with your healthcare requirements and budget.

The example provided in Figure 9-2 highlights the trade-offs involved in selecting a Medicare Advantage plan. It emphasizes the importance of considering both drug coverage and medical benefits when making your decision.

The analysis of the different plans and their associated costs helps to narrow down your choices and allows you to focus on the two or three options that best meet your needs. By weighing the pros and cons of each plan and considering the trade-offs, you can make a more informed and confident decision.

This process of comparing and evaluating competing options is indeed valuable. It helps you prioritize what matters most to you, whether it's affordable drug coverage, comprehensive medical benefits, or a balance between the two. Ultimately, the goal is to select a plan that aligns with your specific healthcare needs and provides the best overall value.

With the information gathered through this analysis, you are now better equipped to make a final decision and choose the Medicare Advantage plan that suits you best.

Choosing the Medicare Advantage Plan

Having all your information organized and comparing Medicare Advantage plans side by side can significantly clarify your options and make the decision-making process easier. Printing out the details of the plans that interest you or using tables like the ones provided in Figures 9-1 and 9-2 can be helpful for visualizing and comparing key details.

However, the Plan Finder does not tell you whether or not your preferred physicians and hospitals accept the plans you're looking at. This data may be crucial in helping you make important choices.

I will show you where to look for the solution to this pressing topic in the next chapters. I will provide pointers on how to determine the network of doctors and hospitals associated with each plan and offer advice on enrolling in a Medicare Advantage plan. Additionally, I will explain the process of switching out of a plan if you change your mind or your circumstances change.

By considering this additional factor alongside the medical benefits, drug coverage, and costs, you can make a well-rounded decision and choose a Medicare Advantage plan that not only meets your healthcare needs but also allows you to access the healthcare providers you prefer.

Which providers accept the plans you're considering

The question of which doctors and hospitals accept the Medicare Advantage plans you're considering is indeed crucial. If you have established relationships with specific healthcare providers and want to continue seeing them, it's important to ensure that the insurance plans you're considering include those providers in their network. On the other hand, if you have experienced difficulties in finding doctors recently, you may prioritize a plan that offers a broad network of providers.

To determine which doctors and hospitals are included in the network of a Medicare Advantage plan, you can take the following steps:

1. Visit the Medicare Plan Finder website and go to the "Benefits & costs" section of any plan you're interested in. Look for the "View Provider Network Directory" link, which will provide you with a list of healthcare providers participating in that plan.

2. Contact each plan directly and request them to mail you a provider list or provide access to a website where you can find their network of providers. This information will give you an idea of which doctors and hospitals are part of their network.

3. Make contact with your primary care physician's office, any specialists you see, and the hospitals you now frequent. Inquire with the insurance billing department about whether or not they accept the Medicare Advantage plans you're interested in. Your selected healthcare providers' approval of the plans may be verified via this transparent channel of communication.

By performing these steps, you can gather the necessary information to assess whether the Medicare Advantage plans you're interested in align with your preferred doctors and hospitals. This will help you make an informed decision that ensures continuity of care and access to the healthcare providers you trust.

Confirming that healthcare providers listed in a plan's network actually accept the plan is an essential step in the process. Simply relying on a plan's claim that a specific doctor is in its network may not provide accurate information. Therefore, it's crucial to take the time to verify this information independently.

Despite updates made to make the Medicare Plan Finder easier to use, some users have reported issues such as incorrect pricing, incorrect lists of covered prescriptions, incorrect doses, and difficulties sorting and storing search results. These problems were observed throughout the 2020 enrollment period for both new and current enrollees. Medicare responded to these complaints by allowing beneficiaries to switch plans if required due to inaccurate information provided by the Plan Finder.

Given these potential inaccuracies, it's important to double-check the information provided by the Plan Finder and independently verify that the healthcare providers you're interested in do indeed accept the specific Medicare Advantage plan you're considering. This ensures that you have the most up-to-date and accurate information when making your enrollment decision. This notification allows patients to be informed of any potential modifications to the provider network and gives them time to make necessary adjustments to their healthcare arrangements if needed. Keeping track of any notifications from your plan and staying informed about changes to the provider network can help ensure that you are aware of any modifications that may affect your access to specific doctors.

Registering in a Medicare Advantage plan

It's time to choose on a plan after you've examined your options and found those that include your chosen physicians and facilities. This choice should reflect your own tastes and the results of your investigation into the various options. If you are having trouble deciding between two or more options, a counselor from your state's SHIP may give helpful insight and point you in the right direction. In Appendix A, you'll discover how to get in touch with SHIP.

Enrolling in a plan is a simple process and can be done through options given below:

1. Click on the "Enroll" button on the Medicare Plan Finder to select your desired plan.
2. Call Medicare's help line at 800-633-4227 (TTY 877-486-2048).
3. The third step is to enroll in the plan by contacting the company directly via its website or phone line.

During the first enrollment period, Medicare recipients who are new to the program may sign up for a Medicare Advantage plan. During the special enrollment period, you may sign up for Medicare Part B even if you waited over the age of 65. Open enrollment runs annually from October 15th to December 7th, and is your best chance to enroll in a plan or make a change.

If you change your views

If you register in a Medicare Advantage health plan and later discover that you are not satisfied with it, there are options available to make changes. Here are several scenarios and the corresponding actions you can take:

1. If you want to switch from an MA plan to traditional Medicare:
   - Each year, between January 1 and February 14, you may take advantage of the annual disenrollment period. You are free to leave your MA plan and return to original Medicare during this grace period.
   - During this time, you may change from your existing MA plan to a separate Part D drug plan if it offers prescription drug coverage.
2. If you signed up for a Medicare Advantage plan when you turned 65:
   - The first year is treated as a trial by Medicare. You have the option to leave your MA plan and return to Original Medicare with a separate Part D medication plan during the first 12 months of coverage.
   - Within the first 63 days after your MA plan coverage ends, you are eligible to enroll in a Medigap insurance.
3. If you're switching to an MA plan for the first time after previously having a Medigap coverage:
   - During the first 12 months of your plan, you have the option to go back to original Medicare and have your Medigap coverage restored.
4. If you receive Extra Help:
   - At any moment throughout the year, you may transfer to a different MA health plan or to original Medicare with a separate Part D medication coverage.

5. If you move outside your plan's service area:
    - You may either switch to a new MA plan in your new location, or revert to original Medicare and a separate Part D medication coverage.
    - You have the legal right to buy a Medigap insurance with the full federal protections if you do so within 63 days after your MA plan coverage expires.
6. If you are admitted to or discharged from a hospital, skilled nursing facility, or similar facility:
    - During your stay in the facility, or up to two months after you leave, you have the option to convert from your current MA plan to another MA plan, or to regular Medicare with a separate Part D medication coverage.
7. If you are a long-term care resident at a nursing home:
    - Anytime throughout the year, you may switch to a new MA plan or to original Medicare with a separate Part D medication coverage.
8. The best possible Medicare Advantage plan is a five-star plan, if one is offered where you live:
    - You are free to make the change at any point throughout the year.
9. If you joined a Medicare Cost plan:
    - You may choose to leave the plan at any time and return to original Medicare at no cost to you.
    - You may switch to a separate Part D drug plan if you have drug coverage under the plan.

These options provide flexibility and opportunities to make changes to your Medicare Advantage plan when certain circumstances arise. For more information and detailed explanations.

Chapter 9

Discovering the Ins and Outs of Specific Medicare Benefits

IN THIS CHAPTER

» Understanding Medicare Part A

» Exploring Medicare's Part B

» Dissecting the Medicare Drug Program

It's commendable that you have taken the initiative to explore and understand the finer points of Medicare coverage. Medicare can be a complex program, and it's not uncommon for individuals to encounter unique situations or questions that require further investigation.

You've done yourself and your viewers a service by digging into these issues and consulting with legal experts in government organizations like Medicare and Social Security for guidance. You have been able to throw light on obscure rules and give thoughts on many Medicare difficulties as a result of your experiences and the obstacles presented by readers.

In this chapter, you aim to address some of these lesser-known aspects of Medicare coverage that may not be adequately explained in official guides. While not everyone may encounter these specific issues, having access to this information empowers individuals to navigate their coverage more effectively and avoid potential pitfalls that may exist within the intricacies of Medicare regulations.

By continuously seeking knowledge and sharing it with others, you contribute to the collective understanding and awareness of Medicare, ensuring that individuals can make informed decisions and maximize the benefits of their coverage.

Examining Part A

Understanding the details of Medicare Part, A is crucial for individuals to fully comprehend the benefits and services it offers. While other chapters in your book provide information on various aspects of Part A, such as coverage, costs, eligibility, and enrollment, this section delves deeper into Part A services.

The notion of hospital benefit periods is addressed in detail here. Individuals may better understand the length of their hospital stay and the extent of their coverage under Part A if this concept is explained. In addition, the section explains other procedures often used in hospitals and SNFs that readers may not be acquainted with but should know about just in case.

By providing insights into these lesser-known aspects of Part A services, you equip readers with the knowledge and understanding needed to navigate potential challenges or unfamiliar practices that may arise during their healthcare journey. It ensures they are well-prepared and informed when dealing with hospitals and SNFs, allowing them to make informed decisions and effectively utilize their Part A benefits.

By including this section in your book, you contribute to readers' overall understanding of Medicare Part A, empowering them to navigate their healthcare experiences with confidence and knowledge.

Being aware of hospital benefit periods

Understanding hospital benefit periods in Medicare can indeed be a complex task. The concept may initially seem straightforward, with a benefit period being perceived as a defined period during which Medicare covers hospital care. However, the actual mechanics of benefit periods differ from this perception.

Officials from Medicare said that a patient's benefit period begins on the first day of hospitalization and concludes after the patient has been discharged for 60 consecutive days. You will still be counted as being within the same benefit period if you are readmitted within 60 days of your earlier discharge. If it has been more than 60 days since your last release and you are readmitted, you will begin a new benefit term. The difference in benefit periods may have a major effect on your out-of-pocket payments, which may add up to a big sum.

Time spent in a skilled nursing facility (SNF) is considered part of the benefit period, which adds another layer of complication due to its own restrictions and cost-sharing obligations. It's important to know that whether you're enrolled in original Medicare or a Medicare Advantage (MA) plan, the regulations and cost structures within benefit periods may vary.

In the upcoming parts of your book, you unravel these intricacies and provide a clearer understanding of benefit periods, specifically as they relate to hospital stays and stays in SNFs. By dissecting and explaining the different components and implications of benefit periods, you offer readers valuable insights into how these periods function under both traditional Medicare and MA plans. This knowledge empowers readers to navigate benefit periods effectively, enabling them to make informed decisions and effectively manage their healthcare costs.

Hospital coverage in traditional Medicare

In Medicare, the costs and coverage for hospital care within each separate benefit period are as follows:

1. Days 1 through 60: Until the Part A hospital deductible is met, the first share of expenses will be your responsibility during this time. The Medicare Part A hospital deductible in 2020 is a maximum of $1,408. After this deductible is satisfied, all hospital costs (including room and board and nursing services) are covered for the duration of the benefit term. However, keep in mind that you will still be responsible for paying your Part B co-pays for any medical care you get while in the hospital.
2. Days 61 through 90: From the 61st day through the 90th day of a benefit period, you will be responsible for a daily co-pay. In 2020, the daily co-pay for this period is $352. It doesn't matter whether you've spent more than 60 days in the hospital altogether or if you've been readmitted within the same benefit period.
3. Beyond 90 days: Medicare coverage will vary if your hospital stay is more than 90 days during the same benefit period. During this time, all expenses must be paid for by you. After the 90th day, however, you may utilize any of your 60 available reserve days to continue being covered. The daily copayment for these reserve days is somewhat high, at $704 as of this writing. There is no upper limit on the number of benefit periods that may be accrued. However, a fresh benefit period begins after 60 days outside of the hospital. The increased Part A deductible (another $1,408 in 2020) must be paid if you are readmitted to the hospital after the first 60-day term has passed before Medicare coverage for that benefit period can resume.

Understanding these cost-sharing arrangements within benefit periods is essential for planning and managing your healthcare expenses.

You're right, the terminology around benefit periods can be confusing, especially when there are multiple rules involving a time frame of 60 days. To clarify, here's a breakdown of the different meanings associated with the 60-day time frame:

1. To be eligible for a new benefit term, you must be out of a hospital or skilled care institution for at least 60 days. This implies that you will begin a new benefit period if you are readmitted to the hospital or skilled care facility after having been released and been outside of either for 60 consecutive days.
2. After you've paid your deductible for the year, Medicare will pay for 100 percent of your hospital bills for up to 60 days. Medicare will pay for all of your hospital bills for up to sixty days each benefit period if you've satisfied your Part A deductible for that time.
3. The maximum number of reserve days you may use to prolong Medicare coverage for hospital treatment during one or more benefit periods is 60, and this limit can be used only once. You may extend your hospital stay beyond the standard 90 days with the

help of lifetime reserve days. You have 60 reserve days available to you throughout the course of your life, but the cost each day is greater.

By understanding these distinctions, you can better navigate the complexities of benefit periods and make informed decisions regarding your Medicare coverage. Additionally, as mentioned, Medigap policies can provide additional coverage for hospital stays beyond the 60-day limit and may cover the Part A deductible, offering further financial protection.

Traditional Medicare's Skilled nursing care in

That's correct. When it comes to skilled nursing facility (SNF) care, the cost-sharing structure is different from hospital care. Here's a breakdown of the costs you are responsible for during each phase of an SNF benefit period:

1. Days 1 through 20: During the first 20 days of an SNF benefit period, you will not have to pay anything for your room, board, or nursing care. All of these expenses are covered by Medicare.

2. Days 21 through 100: From day 21 through day 100 of an SNF benefit period, you are responsible for a daily co-pay. In 2020, the daily co-pay amount is $176. The daily co-pay amount applies to each day after the twentieth day, up to and including the hundredth day.

3. Beyond 100 days: Once you surpass 100 days in an SNF benefit period, you are responsible for all costs associated with your SNF care. Medicare coverage ends at this point, and you will need to cover the expenses out-of-pocket or through other means of payment.

It's important to note that these cost-sharing arrangements for SNF care are specific to Medicare coverage under Part A. The coverage and costs may vary if you have a Medicare Advantage (MA) plan instead. Additionally, Medigap policies may provide additional coverage for SNF care, so it's beneficial to review the details of your specific policy to understand the extent of coverage it offers.

Remember that benefit periods for both hospital and SNF care are separate and have their own cost-sharing rules. Understanding these rules can help you plan and manage your healthcare expenses effectively.

Hospital lifetime reserve days cannot be used to extend Medicare coverage in a skilled nursing facility (SNF) beyond 100 days in any one benefit period. Once you reach 100 days in an SNF benefit period, Medicare coverage ends, and you are responsible for all costs.

However, as you pointed out, supplemental insurance, such as Medigap plans, long-term care insurance, Medicaid, or insurance from an employer or union, may be available to pay the cost of SNF care. The amount to which SNF costs are covered by these supplementary insurance choices varies widely. You should check with your plan and research the specifics of your coverage to see whether or not skilled nursing facility (SNF) costs will be paid and, if so, under what conditions.

Medicare Advantage plans cover hospitals and skilled nursing facilities

Medicare Advantage plans, including HMOs and PPOs, use the same benefit periods as traditional Medicare. It's crucial to remember, however, that Medicare Advantage plans may vary widely in their coverage of hospital and skilled nursing facility costs. There might be significant price discrepancies compared to the standard Medicare system.

In most cases, Medicare Advantage plans will not require you to pay a Part A deductible at the beginning of each benefit period. Instead, they may need a daily copayment of $100 to $500 or more for the first several days of hospitalization or skilled nursing care. After this initial period, they may not charge anything for the remainder of the benefit period. It's crucial to review your specific Medicare Advantage plan's coverage documents or contact the plan directly to confirm their rules and the cost associated with a hospital or SNF stay.

Medicare Advantage plans may have different rules and regulations compared to the traditional Medicare program. Being aware of your plan's specific guidelines will help you better understand the costs and coverage for hospital and skilled nursing care.

Remembering the three-day rule

You must remain in a Medicare-approved skilled nursing facility (SNF) for at least three days before Medicare will pay for your treatment if you are enrolled in the original Medicare program. This rule assures that you've been a hospital patient for at least three full days before being transferred to a skilled nursing facility.

It's crucial to note that the three-day requirement includes the day of admission to the hospital but excludes the day of discharge. Medicare considers a "day" only if you are in the hospital at midnight. Time spent in the emergency room is also not counted towards the three-day requirement. Additionally, it's essential to be an official inpatient during those three days and not merely held under observation status, which will be further explained in the section below.

Staff at the SNF are obligated to tell patients that Medicare will not pay for their treatment if they have not satisfied the three day inpatient criteria. You will be given an Advance Beneficiary Notice of Non-Covered Services (ABN) to sign confirming that you are aware of the full financial responsibility for your SNF stay. More information on Medicare potential nonpayment notices (ABNs) may be found in the section labeled "Receiving a notice saying that Medicare may not pay."

Keep in mind that Medicare and you will not be billed for any additional days you spend in the SNF if the SNF fails to provide you this warning and you remain for treatment nevertheless.

The three-day guideline for coverage in an SNF does have two significant caveats, however:

1. Medicare Advantage Plans: The three-day rule is typically not applied to individuals enrolled in Medicare Advantage plans. These plans, such as Health Maintenance Organizations (HMOs) or Preferred Provider Organizations (PPOs), may have their own guidelines and requirements for coverage in an SNF. It's important to review your specific Medicare Advantage plan's documentation or contact the plan directly to understand their rules and coverage for SNF stays.

2. Different Facility Types: Coverage at a nursing home is limited to three days because to the three-day rule. Medicare will pay for your treatment in a rehabilitation hospital or skilled nursing facility under certain circumstances after you leave the hospital. The nature of the institution and the required level of care will determine the specifics of these regulations. Talk to your doctor and Medicare to find out what services they cover at the place you'll be moving to once you leave the hospital.

By understanding these exceptions, you can better navigate the coverage rules and requirements for SNF stays based on your specific circumstances and healthcare plan.

Defining observation status

Being placed in observation status while in the hospital can have significant implications for your Medicare coverage and billing. Here are some key points to understand about observation status:

Outpatient Classification: When you're in observation status, you are considered an outpatient, even though you may be receiving care and staying in a hospital bed. This distinction is important because Medicare Part A coverage for hospital stays applies only to formally admitted inpatients, not outpatient services.

Doctor's Order: The decision to place you in observation status is typically based on your doctor's assessment and their determination that further observation is necessary before deciding whether to admit you as an inpatient or discharge you. It's crucial to communicate with your doctor and understand their reasoning for placing you in observation status.

Effects on Coverage and Costs: Being in observation status means that your hospital services will be billed under Medicare Part B (outpatient services) rather than Part A (inpatient services). This can result in different coverage rules and higher out-of-pocket costs, such as co-pays and deductibles. It's important to review your Medicare coverage and understand how observation status affects your specific plan.

Impact on Skilled Nursing Facility (SNF) Coverage: If you require further care in an SNF after your hospital stay, Medicare requires a three-day inpatient hospital stay to qualify for SNF coverage (as mentioned earlier). However, days spent under observation status do not count towards the three-day requirement, potentially leaving you responsible for SNF costs if you do not meet the requirement.

To avoid unexpected billing charges and coverage gaps, it's crucial to communicate with your healthcare provider, ask questions about your status, and understand the implications of being in observation status. Being proactive can help you make informed decisions and take necessary steps to ensure appropriate coverage and care.

Consequences of being in observation status

Patients on conventional Medicare may be affected financially by the differential between inpatient and observation status. The most important considerations are as follows:

1. Cost Differences: Medicare Part B covers inpatient stays when the patient is considered to be an outpatient under observation status. You won't have to worry about paying the Part A hospital deductible, but you will have to pay a 20% co-pay for all of your medical care. If you need various services while in the hospital, this might increase your out-of-pocket expenses. You will be liable for paying the whole cost of your hospital stay if you are not enrolled in Medicare Part B.

2. Prescription Drug Coverage: In many hospitals, patients under observation status are not allowed to use their own prescription medications. Instead, the hospital supplies the required medications and bills you for the full retail amount, which your Part D or other prescription coverage may not cover. You would have to pay for hospital care out of pocket before your prescription insurance would cover it.

3. Impact on Skilled Nursing Facility (SNF) Coverage: Medicare requires a three-day inpatient hospital stay for coverage of subsequent care in an SNF. If you spend time in observation status during the three-day period, Medicare will not cover your stay in an SNF. This can leave you responsible for the full cost of SNF care. However, it's important to note that Medicare Advantage plans may have different rules regarding the three-day requirement, so it's advisable to check with your specific plan.

4. Extended Observation Periods: Hospitals are not allowed to keep patients in observation status for more than 48 hours (barring exceptional circumstances) under Medicare rules, but some hospitals have kept patients in observation status for much longer, even exceeding 72 hours or 14 days. Because of this, many are worried about the financial burden of SNF care for patients who need it after lengthy observation stays, and some have even taken legal action as a result.

A class action lawsuit and legislative proposals to do away with the three-day limit are two responses to these problems. Changes to the system have also been pushed for by professional associations. It's important to stay informed about your status, communicate with your healthcare provider, and understand the potential financial implications of being placed under observation status during a hospital stay.

As of this writing, neither the case nor any related legislation has been finalized to any major degree. So far, the main difference is that, as of late autumn 2016, Medicare mandates that all hospitals notify patients in observation units that they are not admitted inpatients. Patients should get MOONSs, or Medicare Outpatient Observation Notices, after 24 hours in observation status and no more than 36 hours following admission. However, they do not provide patients with a means of challenging their classification. Changes to the regulations of observation status will be reflected at www.medicareadvocacy.org/medicare-info/observation-status/.

Hospitals and CAHs that serve Medicare patients (including Medicare Advantage members) are now required to use a new notification form (CMS-10611) beginning in April 2020.

Defense against big bills

These are helpful steps to take if you or someone you're advocating for is placed in observation status at a hospital. To review, here are some strategies for mitigating or resolving the financial consequences of being placed on observation:

1. Inquire about your status: If you haven't gotten the Medicare Outpatient Observation Notice (MOON), ask about your status each day you're in the hospital. You should get a message that verifies your current status and explains its broad clinical justification. If you don't get the notification, you may always request it.
2. Consult your doctor: Speak with your own doctor and discuss whether observation status is justified in your case. Ask them to contact the hospital and explain the medical reasons why you should be admitted as an inpatient.
3. Request reconsideration: Ask the hospital doctor to reconsider your case or refer it to the hospital committee responsible for determining patient status.
4. Explore alternative care options: Discuss with your doctor if you qualify for equivalent treatment at home under Medicare's home health benefit or whether there are alternatives, like as care in a rehabilitation hospital, that may be reimbursed if Medicare won't pay for your stay in a skilled nursing facility due to observation status.
5. Appeal Medicare's decision: If you end up paying for the skilled nursing facility yourself and believe it should have been covered by Medicare, you can appeal Medicare's decision. Make a copy of your Medicare Summary Notice highlighting the

SNF charge and send it along with a letter explaining your appeal to the provided address on the notice Recognizing the improvement standard.

Medicare used to allow for the termination of some forms of coverage, including skilled nursing, home health, and physical therapy, if it was determined that the patient's condition was not improving. When deciding whether or not Medicare should continue to cover certain treatments, administrative contractors employed this method, known as the improvement standard.

However, the case of Jimmo v. Sebelius, a class action lawsuit settled in 2013, clarified that the improvement standard should no longer be applied. It was made clear that Medicare coverage should not be denied based on the absence of potential for improvement or restoration. This settlement agreement emphasized that when skilled services are necessary to prevent or slow further deterioration, coverage should not be denied.

If you encounter a situation where the improvement standard is still being applied to you, it's important to be aware of the statement issued by Medicare officials in April 2013, which emphasizes that coverage cannot be denied based on the absence of potential for improvement or restoration. You can refer to Medicare's fact sheet on this topic as official evidence of this policy.

Usable resources for individuals who are facing coverage decisions based on the improvement standard and need guidance on how to navigate the appeals process. These self-help packets are designed to provide information and assistance in filing Medicare appeals to challenge coverage denials.

By accessing the self-help packets on the Center for Medicare Advocacy's website at www.medicareadvocacy.org/take-action/self-help-packets-for-medicare-appeals/, individuals can obtain valuable resources, sample letters, and step-by-step instructions to help them understand their rights and options when it comes to appealing coverage decisions based on the improvement standard.

Premature hospital discharge

"Important Message from Medicare on Your Rights" and the process for requesting an immediate review or expedited decision if you believe the hospital is discharging you too soon. This information is crucial for individuals who feel they need to stay in the hospital or receive ongoing care but are facing discharge.

To summarize the key points:

You have the right to know your rights and what to do if you think you're being released too soon, therefore the hospital must provide you a copy of the "Important Message from Medicare on Your Rights" notice during the first two days of your stay.

A second copy of the message must be sent to patients who stay in the hospital for more than two days after signing the notice.

You have until noon of the first business day after receiving the discharge notice to appeal the decision and request an urgent review or expedited determination by contacting your local Quality Improvement Organization (QIO).

A "Detailed Notice of Discharge" explaining the rationale for the discharge decision must be sent by the hospital no later than noon on the day after the QIO accepts the appeal has begun if you request an urgent review.

The QIO must make a decision within one day of receiving the hospital records.

Within two days of the appeal being filed, a decision from the QIO should be obtained. You'll have to wait it out in the hospital till then.

You won't have to pay for any extra time in the hospital regardless of the results of the QIO review.

In the event that the QIO rules in your favor, Medicare will continue to cover your hospital bill as normal until a new discharge decision is made. All costs incurred after noon on the day you find out about the verdict will be your responsibility.

You have the right to ask the QIO to review their judgment, and they have three days to do so.

Contacting the QIO as soon as possible after receiving the notification is crucial to starting the appeals procedure on time. Your case will be considered and a decision made in the allotted time limit if you follow these steps.

If the hospital makes a mistake

It is indeed concerning that preventable errors, known as never events, can occur in hospitals. These errors include serious mistakes such as wrong-site surgeries, retained surgical instruments, wrong blood transfusions, post-procedure infections, blood clots, and severe bedsores. However, there are measures in place to address these issues and protect patients.

If you experience a preventable error and require readmission to the hospital to rectify the mistake, there is good news. The hospital cannot charge you or Medicare for the treatment during the readmission. Medicare implemented this policy in 2008, refusing to pay for the costs associated with correcting their own mistakes. Previously, hospitals were able to charge patients for additional treatment, which was unfair and illogical.

A hospital readmits you to rectify a severe mistake and then tries to charge you for the extra treatment, which you should oppose. Instead, you could file a complaint with the regional QIO for Medicare in your area. Patients with questions or concerns regarding their care at a hospital may contact a QIO. Visit www.medicare.gov/Contacts/Default.aspx or http://qioprogram.org/contact, or call Medicare at 800-633-4227 (TTY 877-486-2048), and you'll be connected with your area's Quality Improvement Organization (QIO).

Reporting such situations to the proper authorities is essential for ensuring that corrective measures are done and protecting yourself and others from future damage.

Your rights in a skilled nursing facility

It's important to be aware of the rights and protections afforded to residents of skilled nursing facilities (SNFs). Federal and state laws have established various rights to ensure that residents are treated with respect, receive appropriate care, have privacy, can make choices regarding visitors and their finances, and are free from discrimination, abuse, neglect, and unnecessary restraints.

When you enter a SNF, the facility is required to provide you with written information regarding your legal rights and the facility's policies. This information serves to inform you of your rights and empower you to assert them when necessary.

However, it's unfortunate that there have been instances where administrators of some SNFs have provided incorrect information to Medicare patients. To help you navigate such situations and distinguish fact from fiction, it is essential to be knowledgeable about your rights and the relevant legal authority.

By understanding your rights and the appropriate legal framework, you can advocate for yourself or a loved one if you encounter any discrepancies or challenges within a SNF setting. Being informed and prepared empowers you to protect your rights and ensure that you receive the appropriate care and treatment in accordance with the law.

Leaving the SNF

The director of the SNF is wrong to say that Medicare would not pay for the patient to remain there after she attends her grandson's wedding. As long as the patient's health and rehabilitation are not jeopardized, Medicare regulations permit short trips and temporary breaks from the SNF for activities like attending special events, religious services, family celebrations, and even going for a car ride.

According to the Medicare Benefit Policy Manual, leaving a skilled nursing facility for any of these reasons does not establish evidence that the patient is no longer in need of SNF services. According to the policy manual, it is "not appropriate" for the SNF to inform a patient that they may lose coverage if they transfer to another facility.

Medicare coverage for care in a nursing home is based on a 24-hour period that starts at midnight and ends at midnight. If a patient leaves the facility for a few hours but returns before midnight, they will be considered present for the whole day and will not be subject to Medicare fines.

Therefore, the patient should not have had to worry about losing Medicare coverage for her stay in the SNF upon her return if she had been allowed to attend her grandson's wedding, presuming her health and the level of help provided by her family were adequate for the short absence.

If you are not physically present at the SNF by midnight on a given day, Medicare will not reimburse the cost of your care on that day. However, if you are eligible for SNF coverage, you won't have to worry about paying for those days.

Medicare's coverage for stays at SNFs (short for "skilled nursing facilities") start and stop at midnight daily. Medicare will not cover the cost of your skilled nursing facility (SNF) services if you leave and don't return until after midnight. If you continue to fulfill the requirements for SNF coverage, however, you will not be financially liable for those days.

Keep in mind that you'll still need skilled care and have time remaining on your Medicare benefit period in order to qualify for SNF coverage. Assuming you fulfill these conditions, you will not incur any additional costs when you return to the SNF and your coverage will pick up just where it left off.

A bed-hold fee is a cost charged by certain skilled nursing facilities (SNFs) in exchange for keeping your reserved bed available while you are not there to use it. This charge is made so that your room will be waiting for you when you get back. While some establishments may impose such a charge, others may not, and policies might change.

Inquire in advance with the SNF administration about their bed-hold policy if you intend to take a leave of absence from the SNF, particularly if it will be for a prolonged duration or overnight stay. If they are able to hold your reservation and if there are any costs involved, they can let you know.

Whether or whether you should go on a journey outside of your SNF depends on your mental and physical health, as well as the availability of resources to address your requirements while you're gone. Talking to your doctor is a crucial first step in evaluating your health and deciding whether you may temporarily return home.

Finding a happy medium between going on fun outings and maintaining eligibility for SNF care may be challenging. Medicare laws do permit short trips and visits outside the SNF, but extended stays away might raise questions about your continued need for skilled care.

It's also important to think about whether or not the venue you're going can meet your special requirements, such as having wheelchair access or accessible restrooms. Having someone to look out for your health and safety while you're gone is essential.

Maintaining Medicare coverage and access to required care while enjoying the freedom of occasional trips outside the SNF is possible if you follow Medicare standards and consult with your doctor beforehand.

Leaving SNF care (and returning)

Medicare coverage for the patient's time in the SNF would not be voided or altered by a trial visit home. This is the case regardless of whether the patient returns to the SNF or choose to get care at home.

According to Medicare regulations, coverage of earlier SNF treatment is unaffected by a trial visit home. If the patient continues to fulfill the Medicare criteria for skilled care, their eligibility and coverage for the days they were in the SNF will not change.

Getting in touch with Medicare or talking to Medicare lawyers is a good idea if the SNF refuses to accept Medicare as payment in order to safeguard the patient's rights and Medicare coverage.

Medicare coverage will not change if you need to return to the SNF after a trial stay at home or for any other reason. Medicare coverage may be reinstated if you return to a skilled nursing facility (the same one or a different one) within 30 days, rather than requiring a fresh qualifying 3-day hospital stay as an admitted patient.

Medicare will continue to pay for your skilled nursing facility (SNF) treatment if you return there within 30 days, as long as you've already spent at least three days in a hospital.

Medicare will pay for skilled nursing facility treatment if you need it, but only if you enter an SNF within 30 days after leaving the hospital.

In order to have a seamless transition and to fully grasp the Medicare coverage criteria and regulations that apply to your case, it is essential that you speak with both your healthcare physician and the SNF.

Doctor of your choice

The statement made by the SNF staff members in Florida is false. According to Medicare officials, the claim that bringing in a primary-care physician (PCP) would result in the loss of Medicare coverage for the stay in the skilled nursing facility (SNF) is unfounded and contradicts the requirements for SNFs participating in the Medicare program.

Medicare regulations do not restrict the type of healthcare provider that can be consulted while in an SNF. Medicare beneficiaries have the right to choose and consult with their own PCP or any other healthcare professional of their choice. This includes receiving visits from a PCP while staying in an SNF.

It's important to be aware of your rights as a Medicare beneficiary and to communicate any concerns or issues regarding access to healthcare providers with the SNF administration. Medicare officials can also provide guidance and support if you encounter any difficulties in exercising your rights.

The Code of Federal Regulations, specifically Section 483.10 (d) under "Free Choice," establishes the rights of individuals in skilled nursing facilities and long-term care nursing homes. According to this regulation, residents have the following legal rights:

1. The right to choose a personal attending physician: You have the right to select a physician who will be responsible for your care while you are in the facility.
2. The right to be fully informed about your care and treatment: You have the right to receive complete and accurate information about your care, including any proposed changes that may affect your well-being. This ensures that you have the necessary information to make informed decisions about your health.
3. The right to participate in planning your care and treatment: Unless you are deemed incompetent or incapacitated under the laws of your state, you have the right to actively participate in decisions regarding your care and treatment. This means being involved in the planning process and having a say in any changes made to your care.

These rights are in place to protect your autonomy and ensure that you are actively involved in decisions related to your health and well-being while residing in a skilled nursing facility or long-term care nursing home.

If Medicare refuses to pay, you may still submit a claim

If you find yourself in a situation where skilled nursing facility (SNF) staff tells you that Medicare may not cover a specific service or your entire stay, but you are unsure whether they are correct, here's what you can do:

Request an Advance Beneficiary Notice of Non-Coverage (ABN): If the SNF staff believes that Medicare may not cover a particular service or your stay, they should provide you with an ABN. This notice informs you of the potential non-coverage and gives you the opportunity to make an informed decision. To learn more about your choices and next actions after receiving an ABN, see "Receiving a notice saying that Medicare may not pay."

You have the legal right to require the SNF to submit a claim for Medicare coverage on your behalf to the regional Medicare contractor. The contractor may make a final judgment about whether or not the service will be covered using this method, known as demand billing.

Exercise your right to appeal: You have the option to file an appeal if your claim is rejected. You may appeal the refusal and try to have the service covered via this method.

It's important to remember that if you receive a service that is later determined not to be covered by Medicare, you will be responsible for paying the SNF for that service out-of-pocket. However, during the time you are waiting for the contractor's decision regarding Part A coverage (such as your stay in the facility), the SNF cannot request payment.

Don't simply accept the SNF's statement as the final decision on coverage. By following the steps above, you can ensure that the official coverage decision is made by Medicare and retain your right to appeal if necessary.

Part B

Medicare Part B covers a vast variety of medical treatments and supplies, making it difficult to understand. You may check with Medicare or your healthcare provider ahead of time to find out whether or not a certain service or product will be reimbursed, as well as any associated fees. If you want Medicare to fund a treatment or purchase, you should do everything you can to make sure it is considered medically essential. Medicare allows you to get a second opinion from a different doctor if you're worried about the diagnosis or treatment they've given you. It may be necessary to submit a claim to Medicare on your own in rare circumstances, such as if your provider refuses to submit a claim or if you obtain treatment outside of the United States. These rules apply only to the original Medicare program; for information about your particular coverage under a Medicare Advantage plan, please contact your company directly.

Will Medicare will insure your treatment

Determining whether Medicare will cover a specific medical service can be a bit complex. While many assume that coverage is a straightforward "yes" or "no" for all Medicare beneficiaries across the country, it depends on various factors, including your location.

National Coverage Determinations (NCDs) and Local Coverage Determinations (LCDs) are the two types of Medicare coverage. National Coverage Determinations (NCDs) outline the medical treatment and supplies that Medicare will pay for and under what circumstances. These NCDs apply to all Medicare recipients throughout the country. Medicare Parts A and B claim processors, known as Medicare Administrative Contractors (MACs), are responsible for establishing LCDs in their respective regions. Coverage for services not mandated to be paid for by NCDs is at the discretion of MACs. Beneficiaries in the contractor's service area (which may span several states) are subject to LCDs.

You may use one of many methods to determine whether Medicare will pay for a certain treatment. If you have questions regarding Medicare coverage, you may contact Medicare directly. If you contact Medicare and your treatment isn't on their lists of covered services, they may ask you to get the correct billing code from your provider and call back so they may look into it.

One alternative is to talk to the doctor or expert who will be doing the procedure. If they don't know, they may ask their local MAC or look it up in the Medicare Coverage Database.

It's important to remember that the Medicare website (www.medicare.gov/coverage/your-medicare-coverage.html) could include some coverage information, but it might not be all-inclusive or contain LCDs that apply to your particular location. All NCDs and LCDs are available in the Medicare Coverage Database (www.cms.gov/medicare-coverage-database/), which allows for more in-depth searches but is mainly intended for healthcare professionals and may be difficult for consumers to access.

Warning that Medicare coverage may not be available

You are more likely to be informed if the healthcare treatment you need is not guaranteed to be covered by Medicare. An ABN may be issued by any medical service provider if they feel Medicare would not cover the cost of providing the service. This includes doctors, hospitals, labs, nursing homes, home health agencies, medical equipment suppliers, and ambulance services. An ABN alerts you to the possibility that you may be financially accountable for anything.

There is one single scenario in which you will almost surely obtain an ABN when you call for an ambulance. Keep in mind that not all service providers must provide an ABN. However, an ABN is often issued by ambulance services because to the possibility that Medicare may not pay the costs involved. You may then decide whether or not to continue with the service, bearing the risk of any associated charges, based on this heads-up regarding the possibility of non-coverage.

ABN - Advance Beneficiary Notice

An ABN might ask you to sign it after reviewing three options which are as:

- You want the service or product being offered, and Medicare should be billed for it. You acknowledge, however, that you will be on the hook for payment if Medicare opts not to reimburse the expense. If you disagree with Medicare's judgment, you may file an appeal.
- You're interested in the service or product, but Medicare payments should not be included. You, on the other hand, agree to cover the entire price of the service or product. Because you will be opting out of Medicare coverage, you will not have the chance to subsequently challenge Medicare's decision.
- You do not want the service or item that is being offered. If you choose this option, you will not have to pay for it. However, like option 2, you will not have the opportunity to appeal Medicare's decision since you have decided not to receive the service or item.

In simple terms, ABN asks you to decide whether you want the service or item and how you would like to handle the payment. Depending on your choice, you may or may not be able to appeal Medicare's decision regarding coverage.

Since ABN does not influence whether Medicare would pay the treatment or goods, consumer advocates often suggest going with the first choice. This is because it lets you maintain your right according to the appeal. After examining your application for Medicare coverage, they may still decide to do so.

It's possible, however, that you'll feel some anxiety at the prospect of having to pay the full amount out of pocket if Medicare decides to deny the claim. The projected price for the service should be included on the ABN form so the customer may make a well-informed choice.

If you choose with option one, your provider may refuse to pay, and your healthcare provider can demand payment up advance. If Medicare does not pay the whole amount, the provider may retain the remainder. Note that Medicare Part B claims may be processed in a different way than Part A claims and be subject to various regulations.

Choosing option one, in other words, lets you preserve your appeal rights and provides Medicare another chance to change their mind. But if Medicare doesn't pay, you could have to pay the whole thing out of pocket, and the provider can retain the cash even if Medicare eventually decides to reject the claim.

As I tend to explain in the earlier section "Knowing your rights in a skilled nursing facility," you can't be asked to pay for a Part A service specifically when your claim is being in consideration. If Medicare approves coverage, either initially or after an appeal, the provider must provide a reimbursement within 30 days, less any applicable deductibles or copayments.

It is advised that you use the first option on the ABN form if you have supplemental insurance, such as job benefits, that covers expenses not paid for by Medicare. This is crucial if you require evidence of a Medicare refusal in order to make use of the supplementary insurance.

However, if your supplementary insurance is a Medigap policy, it will not pay for any expenses associated with a Part B treatment that Medicare does not. Medigap plans are meant to complement Original Medicare, not to pay for the costs that Original Medicare does not.

Ambulance services

If you call an ambulance, then there is a high probability that you will be given an ABN. Simply dialing 911 does not guarantee automatic coverage with Medicare. Moreover, the conditions for Medicare coverage for ambulance services are quite strict. Generally, Medicare will cover the ambulance services only if you are transported to the nearest facility which can provide the necessary care, while meeting other coverage conditions. Additionally, at least one of the following coverage conditions should be true:

- Your health is rapidly deteriorating, and you need immediate medical attention. This includes but is not limited to states of unconsciousness, shock, bleeding, extreme agony, and the need for medical attention en route.
- Taking a different mode of transportation might be harmful to your health. In the absence of an imminent danger, however, this requirement may be satisfied only if you have a formal order from your doctor prohibiting the use of any other mode of transportation.
- Because you are either in a distant area or stuck in traffic, land transportation to where you need to go would take too long, and you thus need to be carried by air ambulance or helicopter.

The definition of an ambulance is regulated by Medicare itself: A stretcher and other medical equipment, as well as personnel qualified to provide first aid, are essential components of each ambulance. Therefore, wheelchair accessible vehicles do not fall within Medicare's coverage guidelines.

If you fulfill Medicare's requirements for coverage, the program's Part B will cover the cost of your ambulance ride, leaving you liable for 20 percent of the total (unless you have Medigap or another kind of supplementary insurance that covers your portion).

If the paramedics determine that you do not qualify, they will issue you an ABN with the same choices detailed above.

Ambulance services are allowed to request payment in advance (before transport), with the promise of a refund if Medicare ultimately agrees to cover the cost.

For more details, see "Medicare Coverage of Ambulance Services" at www.medicare.gov/Pubs/pdf/11021-Medicare-Coverage-of-Ambulance-Services.pdf.

Find out a service's cost in advance

It is understandable to have concerns about the out-of-pocket costs associated with a specific treatment or procedure, particularly when it involves major surgery or is expected to be expensive. However, obtaining a precise answer in advance regarding the exact out-of-pocket expenses can be challenging.

Several factors contribute to the difficulty of determining upfront costs. Firstly, medical procedures and treatments vary in complexity, and the overall cost may depend on individual circumstances and the specific details of the procedure. Additionally, healthcare providers often need to consider various factors such as insurance coverage, deductibles, copayments, and the negotiated rates with insurers, which can differ based on the specific insurance plan.

the issue of ambiguity in healthcare costs extends beyond Medicare and applies to various insurance plans. The variability in charges for the same treatment or procedure can be significant, even among different hospitals or doctors.

Medicare Part B's payment system adds another layer of uncertainty. In the traditional Medicare program, Medicare pays 80% of the "Medicare-approved" amount for services covered under Part B, while the remaining 20% is the patient's responsibility. However, the specific amount or calculation of that 20% can be unclear because Medicare bases its payments on geographical variations in local medical costs.

This means that the "Medicare-approved" amount, which Medicare uses to determine its portion of the payment, can vary depending on the location where the service is provided. As a result, your out-of-pocket share of the cost may fluctuate based on the specific payment rates and medical costs in your area.

It is important to note that private insurance plans may also have similar arrangements, where the patient's share is determined by a percentage of the allowed amount or a negotiated rate specific to the plan and the provider.

To gain a better understanding of your financial responsibility, it is advisable to reach out to your healthcare provider, hospital, or insurance company for more specific cost information. They can provide estimates or explanations regarding the expected out-of-pocket expenses for a particular treatment or procedure based on your insurance coverage and the rates negotiated with providers in your area. Additionally, reviewing your insurance policy documents or contacting your insurance provider's customer service can offer insights into the payment structure and cost-sharing details of your specific plan.

So, what do you have to choose from? Inquire about the cost of the procedure and whether or not Medicare will cover it from the surgeon or other specialist providing your treatment. Another option is to get in touch with the hospital's billing department. When preparing for surgery, keep in mind that no one can tell you an exact number since they just don't know what will happen until you're already in the operating room. Additional specialists (such an anesthesiologist) may be billed at their own rates in addition to the surgeon's fees.

Maximizing your coverage

It is important to understand that even if Medicare generally covers a specific service, there may still be conditions that apply to individual cases. These conditions are not specific to an individual beneficiary but are part of the overall Medicare coverage guidelines.

For beneficiaries enrolled in Medicare Advantage plans, these conditions are typically outlined in the evidence of coverage documents provided by the plan. However, for those enrolled in traditional Medicare, such documents are not provided. Therefore, it is crucial to be aware of the conditions within the program and act accordingly to avoid disappointment, frustration, and potentially unnecessary expenses.

Here are some key considerations regarding Medicare conditions:

1. Doctor participation and assignment: When visiting a doctor for the first time, it is essential to inquire if they accept Medicare and if they accept assignment. Accepting assignment means that the doctor agrees to accept the Medicare-approved amount as full payment for services. This information is crucial as it can impact on your costs and coverage. For example, certain preventive tests that Medicare covers for free are only free when obtained from a doctor who accepts assignment.

2. Approved providers: Use of Medicare-approved providers is required for beneficiaries to obtain coverage for skilled nursing or rehabilitation care, home health services, dialysis therapy, or medical equipment and supplies. Medicare won't help you pay for treatments from non-approved providers. Medicare's website or calling Medicare directly will supply you with a list of authorized providers, often known as contract suppliers.

3. Coverage intervals: Medicare establishes limitations on the frequency of coverage for certain routine tests, especially preventive screenings that are offered free of charge. For instance, mammograms for breast cancer screening are typically covered once every 12 months, while cardiovascular screenings to detect heart attack and stroke risks are covered every five years. By familiarizing yourself with these conditions and adhering to them, you can better navigate Medicare coverage and avoid unexpected costs or denied services. If you have further questions or need specific information regarding coverage conditions, contacting Medicare directly or referring to the official Medicare resources can provide valuable guidance.

Specific About the Service You Want

If the provider or the doctor misinterprets your request, you may wind up paying for a treatment that Medicare doesn't cover. For example, Medicare's wellness visit plan includes yearly checks at no cost to the participant. You'll get a chance to talk to the doctor about how you're feeling, and they'll check vitals like your blood pressure and weight. However, the wellness visit is not the same as the annual physical that both physicians and patients often discuss. Therefore, Medicare will not reimburse a physical exam if you opt for one instead of a wellness checkup.

Other Requirements

Medicare coverage of a certain service may be subject to additional requirements. To get home health care, for instance, you must be unable to leave your house (homebound) and have your doctor sign a form stating that you need this service. Moreover, in order to get medical equipment, your physician will need to submit a certificate of medical necessity.

Your Right to Second Opinions

It's natural to be concerned about making the appropriate option while facing a non-emergency surgery or any significant operation. It's crucial to understand that Medicare will reimburse the expense of speaking with another doctor if you want a second or even third opinion.

Waiting for a second opinion is not recommended in an emergency situation where your health or life is in jeopardy. However, for elective operations or other significant procedures that are not life-threatening, you can take your time considering your treatment options.

If you have traditional Medicare and want a second opinion from a different specialist, you may request a referral from your primary care physician. You might even consult with a different expert if you like.

Medicare will pay for a third medical opinion if the first two are contradictory. Twenty percent of the Medicare-approved Part B cost will be your responsibility in these situations. This is the case if you see a doctor that accepts patients with Medigap or similar additional insurance. If you get a second or third opinion, or decide not to have the treatment at all, the choice of doctor to carry it out is still yours to choose.

If you're enrolled in a Medicare Advantage plan, you still have the freedom to seek out other perspectives. To get a second or third opinion from a doctor in the plan's network, you may require a referral from your primary care physician in many plans, especially HMOs. In addition, the co-pays or fees associated with these appointments may be different than what you'd pay with traditional Medicare.

Filing a claim with Medicare

Most healthcare services are covered by Medicare without your having to contact Medicare directly. Instead, Medicare will be billed by the doctor or healthcare provider, and Medicare will pay their portion. Medicare's coordination of benefits system will automatically send your claim to your secondary insurer (such as Medigap or employer-sponsored insurance) if you have any. There are, however, two instances in which you must submit a claim promptly if you have conventional Medicare.

Doctor does not file a claim

Individuals contacting Medicare directly for payment purposes is extremely rare. All healthcare providers, including doctors, hospitals, labs, and medical equipment suppliers, are legally required to submit claims to Medicare on behalf of the people they serve under the traditional Medicare program. It is crucial to understand that providers that have opted out of Medicare cannot bill Medicare for your treatment, and you cannot bill Medicare directly either. Doctors and providers who are enrolled in a Medicare Advantage plan should send their bills to the appropriate plan.

In the rare circumstance that a provider is unable or unwilling to bill Medicare for your treatment, you have the option of filing your own claim. To assure Medicare payment, all claims must be submitted within 12 months of the date of service, whether from the provider or by yourself. As a result, it's a good idea to verify your Medicare Summary Notices frequently to confirm that all of your medical appointments, tests, and treatments are accurately documented, suggesting that the claims were properly and promptly submitted. If any claims are missing, you should request that they be filed by the provider. If it fails, you will need to file a claim with Medicare directly.

The CMS-1490S form is used to submit a claim to Medicare and comes with instructions on how to complete it and where to send it. Medicare's help line may be reached at 800-633-4227 (TTY 877-486-2048), and the form can be downloaded in both English and Spanish at www.cms.gov/Medicare/CMS-Forms/CMS-Forms-Items/CMS012949. Please provide a detailed invoice for the services you provided.

Medicare to deny a claim

Having Medicare withhold payment may seem counterintuitive. Medicare is the principal insurer, therefore if you have secondary insurance like retiree benefits, your insurer may need to formally reject the service or treatment before they would pay for it.

You must provide a copy of the Medicare denial letter to your secondary insurer if you get a formal rejection after receiving an Advance Beneficiary Notice of Non-Coverage (as stated above). Even if Medicare hasn't officially denied your claim, you may still submit the CMS-14908 form (see above) to get reimbursed. Simply filing a claim to Medicare for payment of a particular medical treatment initiates the reimbursement process. You may ask your secondary insurer to reconsider Medicare's decision to deny payment by sending them a copy of the rejection letter Medicare provides you.

Part D

Prescription drugs purchased by patients outside of a hospital setting are covered by Medicare Part D. Medication that you purchase and administer yourself, as opposed to medical care administered at a clinic or hospital.

In this piece, we'll take a closer look at Medicare's coverage for pharmaceuticals. What to do if your Medicare Part D plan doesn't pay for your medicines or limits your ability to get them is something we'll go into later. In addition, we will detail why some drugs have lower co-pays than others, how to avoid the coverage gap known as the "doughnut hole," where to get the shingles vaccine, and highlight a no-cost service that can help you deal with the potential side effects of taking multiple medications.

It's important to remember that this section applies equally to Part D coverage acquired via a Medicare Advantage plan and a stand-alone prescription plan.

How a plan may restrict your drug coverage

It is essential to be aware that no Medicare Part D plan provides coverage for every medication. If you find out that your plan doesn't pay for one or more of your drugs, you may have options. However, it may be annoying to be told by the pharmacist that your insurance company needs prior authorization before covering a prescription you know is on the formulary (the list of authorized drugs). What is happening in these situations?

This occurs due of the limitations imposed by Part D. Next, we'll talk about the many kinds of limitations you can encounter and how to circumvent them, how to get an exemption from your doctor, and where to find the correct kind of medical professional to write you a prescription.

Prior authorization, quantity limits, and step therapy

Prior authorization, quantity limitations, and step therapy are among usage management methods that Medicare Part D insurers may employ to control costs. However, those who must cope with these limitations may see them as substantial hurdles to jump before their prescription drugs are covered by their plan. Now, let's examine these limitations in more detail:

- **Prior authorization:** Certain medications may require prior authorization under a Part D plan. This restriction is often enforced when the drug is potent and poses possible safety risks if used incorrectly or for an extended period. To get this restriction lifted, your doctor must state that the medicine is medically necessary. They must provide you with convincing explanations of why you need the drug. Furthermore, if your drug is occasionally covered under Part B (medical insurance), the plan may require information from your doctor to determine whether it should be covered under Part B or Part D.
- **Quantity limits:** Medicare Part D coverage does not end suddenly after a certain amount of time, unlike what certain advertisements may lead you to believe. These phrases, on the other hand, imply that your doctor has prescribed a more intensive course of treatment than is typical under your plan. If your doctor prescribes a drug that you need to take twice daily, but the standard dosage is only once, your insurance company may refuse to pay for it unless your doctor can provide evidence that the double dosage is necessary for your treatment.
- **Step therapy:** Step therapy is a kind of restriction in Medicare Part D. This means that your plan needs you to try cheaper drugs identical to the one prescribed by your doctor before considering coverage for the more expensive prescription. To get around this restriction, your doctor must show that you have tried lower-cost medications but found them to be less successful in treating your medical condition than the prescription medication.

While it may be logical to think that all Part D plans to implement the same drug restrictions based on a uniform Medicare policy, the reality is considerably different. In fact, each plan is free to choose which drugs in its formulary are subject to one or more restrictions. This technique may look arbitrary, but it can provide you with more options to locate alternate alternatives and receive necessary prescriptions while avoiding burdensome regulations.

This personalized approach by plans enables flexibility and various workarounds to navigate the system efficiently.

You may be able to avoid issues with prescription limits or lack of coverage by:

- **Trying another drug:** It's possible that your Medicare Part D plan has other medications on its formulary that can treat your medical condition successfully while being less expensive. It's advisable to discuss this option with your doctor, as they can advise you on if switching to a different drug, such as a generic or older medication, could drastically lower your drug costs.
- **Trying another plan:** Since different Part D plans place different limitations on, or don't cover at all, certain medications, you may move to a different plan during open enrollment if your current one does.

Exception with your doctor's Help

If switching to another drug or Part D plan is not an option, you can still seek coverage for the medication prescribed by your doctor through your current Medicare Part D plan. To address this need, Medicare law established a process called "requesting an exemption" or a "coverage determination."

Although you may not be able to change your medicine or switch plans at this time, you can contact your existing plan and request that they waive their restrictions and offer coverage for the medication prescribed by your doctor. You can manage the guidelines specified in Medicare law and argue for the coverage you seek by completing the exception process.

Requesting an exemption includes formally speaking with your plan and explaining why receiving the prescription drug is medically required, regardless of any existing limits or restrictions. Based on the facts provided, the plan will examine your request and make a coverage determination.

Understanding this option and using the exception process might be critical in ensuring that you have access to the required medication under your existing Part D coverage. By using Medicare's coverage determination procedure, you can address your specific healthcare needs and verify that the prescribed drug is properly covered.

Remember that knowing your rights and investigating your alternatives allows you to take an active role in managing your healthcare and maximizing the benefits provided by Medicare Part D.

It is critical to have the assistance of your doctor or someone representing you when filing an exemption request for drug coverage. In fact, without your doctor's supporting statement, the plan may not give your request adequate attention or may cause delays in the process. Let's look at how this procedure works:

- You may save yourself time and frustration by having your prescribing doctor handle the submission of your Part D exemption request on your behalf. Nurse practitioners and physician assistants are examples of other competent healthcare professionals who may make a request on your behalf. You may either have them call your plan and make the request or provide them with the necessary forms. They, or you, may also access the necessary paperwork on the CMS website (www.cms.gov). Changes were made to Parts C and D, Enrollee Grievance, Organization/Coverage Determinations, and Appeals Guidance, to account for new regulations that will go into effect on January 1, 2020. If you need to access the updated form, it may be found at www.cms.gov/Medicare/Appeals-and-Grievances/MedPrescriptDrugApplGriev.
- Within 72 hours of receiving your doctor's supporting statement, your Part D plan is required to react under Medicare guidelines. It is important to remember that the hours used here are not business hours but rather real hours. Your doctor may ask for a fast-track exemption if waiting the standard 72 hours would be dangerous to your health or life. In such a case, the plan must react within 24 hours, again in real time.
- In most cases, authorized exceptions are effective until the end of the fiscal year. However, the plan may necessitate more frequent requests for some prior authorization restrictions. If this is the case, you and your doctor will have to go through the same process again, possibly numerous times during the year.
- If your Part D plan denies your request for an exception, you may appeal the decision by seeking a reconsideration. This entails asking the plan to reconsider its decision. You can escalate the dispute to higher levels of appeal if necessary. It's worth noting that you can take these procedures not just in the event of denial but also if your plan fails to reply within the time frames indicated.

Prescriptions from the right doctor

Medicare requires Part D plans to deny coverage for medicines issued by non-Medicare providers or providers who have officially withdrawn from Medicare. This regulation was enacted to prevent the dispensing of illicit prescriptions and to bar doctors whose licenses have been revoked or who have a history of patient complaints.

In reality, this rule applies to very few doctors and nurses. If this is the case, however, you should know that Medicare stipulates that you get a three-month supply of the Part D-covered drug ordered. You have the choice of seeing a different doctor or waiting three months to allow the current one time to join or leave Medicare.

Grappling with the tier system of co-pays

Few things upset Part D members more than unexpected increases in their drug co-pays. It's reasonable that readers are surprised and frustrated when prices rise significantly from one month to the next. In one situation, a reader voiced concern about a generic prescription that increased from a $5 co-pay to a whopping $45 co-pay. This type of shift is unacceptable, but it's worth noting the timing. The co-pay increase occurred during the changeover from December to January, when plans are free to change their fees. In this case, the plan merely shifted the individual's medication from one pricing bracket to another. Part D price ranges will be covered in full in the following sections.

Pricing Tiers?

Part D plans categorize different types of drugs using pricing tiers, which determine the co-pays charged for each tier. As a result, some medications may be more expensive than others. The pricing tiers are as follows:

- **Tier One:** Since the plan's suggested generic pharmaceuticals are the most cost-effective options, they make up Tier 1, which has the lowest co-pay.
- **Tier Two:** Prescription drugs in the second tier have a moderate copay since they are well-liked branded brands. Brand-name drugs are those without an equivalent, less expensive generic version.
- **Tier three:** Compared to the previous tiers, this tier has a higher co-pay because it covers the plan's non-preferred brand-name drugs. These drugs are either too costly or the plan has been unable to negotiate sufficient discounts with the makers.
- **Specialty Tier:** The specialty tier includes drugs that are extremely expensive or highly specialized such as those used for post-organ transplant anti-rejection treatment and some cancer therapies. Because these drugs are typically expensive, Medicare limits the co-pays that plans may charge for them. The co-pay for specialty tier drugs in plans with an annual deductible cannot exceed 25% of the drug's cost, whereas the limit in plans without a deductible is 33%. Even with these percentages, the real amount that individuals may be required to pay can be large.

Some Medicare Part D plans further subdivide their drugs into as many as six distinct categories. Whereas some plans only have one tier and apply the same cost percentage (about 25%) to all covered medications, others have many tiers.

It's vital to remember that the first coverage period is the only time that price levels apply to Part D plans. After you've paid your yearly deductible and before you reach the coverage gap, often known as the "doughnut hole" (if your medication costs surpass a particular level), this is the time frame in which your insurance will begin to pay for 100% of your prescription drug costs.

Find out your plan's pricing tiers?

Each Part D prescription medication plan has its own pricing tier system. As a result, co-pays for the same drug might vary greatly amongst plans. You can use the following approaches to understand the specific tiers and associated costs for your drugs inside a Part D plan:

- Check the formulary on the plan's official website. The formulary lists all the medications covered by the plan, as well as the pricing tier assigned to each drug for the current year. There is also a key or guide inside the formulary that describes the co-pay (a fixed cash amount) or coinsurance (a percentage of the drug's cost) applicable to each tier.
- You may also call your Part D provider to find out what category your medication falls under and how much your co-pay will be. It's crucial to remember that plans might change the coverage of some prescriptions from one year to the next. If you call them in November or December, you may find out what the tiers and co-pays will be in January of the next year.
- Another way to get information on pricing tiers and co-pays for your drugs is to use the Plan Finder tool on Medicare's official website at www.medicare.gov/find-a-plan.To access the details page of the specific plan you are enrolled in or considering, follow the instructions on the website Scroll down this page until you reach the part titled "Drug coverage & costs." You will discover a list of your prescribed drugs and the related tiers and co-pays directly under this category.

To further refine your results, choose your medicine purchasing method (mail order, preferred retail pharmacy, or regular retail pharmacy) from the "Tier Drug Cost for" drop-down option. Choose whether you typically purchase one month's worth or three months' worth of your medications.

Your drugs are suddenly switched to a higher price tier?

As a tactic to balance the expense of keeping relatively low premiums, Part D plans may sometimes transfer a medicine from a lower tier to a higher tier. This change is often made at the beginning of the calendar year, when plans have the most leeway to make adjustments to their fees and benefits. The plan may be able to reduce costs while still covering a prescription if it is moved to a more expensive tier. You should know your rights if a tier change happens throughout the year while you are already taking the medicine.

- Make a formal request to maintain this year's reduced copayment rate. It's possible that your plan will let you remain paying the lower co-pay even if the medicine has been changed to a higher tier without you having to do anything. If this isn't the case, you may ask your insurance company to keep your low co-pay in place. Another option is to request a coverage decision by following the steps mentioned in "Requesting an exception with your doctor's help." Taking these measures will increase the likelihood that you will be able to continue obtaining the prescription at a reduced cost.

You may submit a formulary tier exception request if your doctor prescribes a brand-name medicine that is put in a higher tier on your plan's formulary. Your medication may be transferred to a more affordable pricing tier under this provision. There are, however, requirements that must be completed before this request may be processed. If there are similar medications on the formulary, yours will need to be at a higher tier to be covered. In addition, your physician must write a statement justifying why this medication is the best option for your condition. You can't ask for a medicine in the most expensive category to be switched to a cheaper one, and you can't have a brand-name drug relocated to a generics-only tier.

Changing to a different Part D plan before the new year begins is your only option if your medication is moved to a far more expensive tier. You may prevent the financial effect of a tier shift by switching to a less expensive Part D plan, which can be found by comparing and contrasting various plans.

Doughnut hole

The coverage gap in the Part D program, commonly referred to as the "doughnut hole," has been a well-known and widely disliked aspect of the program. Prior to 2011, individuals who entered the coverage gap had to bear the full cost of their medications out-of-pocket. However, since the passage of the Affordable Care Act (ACA) in 2010, the doughnut hole has been gradually closing each year.

Coverage gaps were expected to be filled up by 2020. However, 2019 budget legislation changed the schedule. Beneficiaries will now be responsible for paying just 25% of the total cost of their medicines during the coverage gap, according to the new regulations. In 2020, the doughnut hole will last until your deductible and copayments total $6,350. When this point is reached, coverage becomes disastrous. For the rest of the calendar year, your sole cost for prescription medicines will be a modest coinsurance or co-payment during this period. The coverage gap occurs during what Medicare calls Phase 3 of the Part D coverage process.

Here is important information regarding the doughnut hole under the Affordable Care Act (ACA):

- Under the Affordable Care Act (ACA), all Part D enrollees are eligible for discounts on prescription drugs if they enter the coverage gap, commonly known as the doughnut hole. However, there is an exception for those receiving Extra Help. Beneficiaries who qualify for Extra Help already receive year-round coverage without experiencing the coverage gap.

- The coverage gap savings may be obtained without submitting an application or completing any paperwork. When you buy your prescriptions from a pharmacy, whether it's a brick-and-mortar store or an online pharmacy, the savings will be applied and removed from your total automatically. Taking advantage of these price reductions requires no more effort on your part.
- You will not get any more time in the coverage gap from the brand-name medicine manufacturers' discounts. However, the amount saved from these reductions does go against your out-of-pocket maximum, allowing you to eventually leave the gap. You should know that these price reductions are not paid for directly by you. However, the restriction does not apply to any brand-name or generic pharmaceuticals for which the government has paid the coverage gap price. It's important to remember that if you want your drugs to count against the limit while you're in the gap, you'll need to buy them via your Part D plan.
- All brand-name medications eligible for coverage under Part D must have manufacturer discounts made available by the manufacturer. This implies that a medicine will not be covered by a Part D plan if the manufacturer does not take part in offering the doughnut hole discounts. Your Medicare Part D plan will not cover the cost of the medication in this very improbable scenario. Check your Part D plan's formulary to be sure the medications you need are included and distributed by manufacturers that are a part of the program.

Drugs that are not normally covered by your plan but have been authorized as an exception because your doctor has requested them are also eligible for the coverage gap reductions under Medicare Part D.

Discounts for the gap period will be applied after any coverage provided by your Part D plan has been deducted from the total cost of the medication.

A minor dispensing charge, usually between $2 and $5, will be added to the cost of your medicine when you pick it up at the pharmacy. You are responsible for this payment in addition to the gap discounts.

In addition to saving Medicare recipients billions of money (an estimated $26 billion since 2010), there has been an intriguing side effect brought about by this modification in the legislation. During the coverage gap, some beneficiaries may actually pay less for some prescriptions than they did earlier in the year when they had full coverage. It's feasible, albeit it may seem impossible at first.

Let's take Brian's situation as an example; his Part D plan required him to pay a $95 co-pay for a high-priced tier brand-name medicine. In 2020, Brian paid just $72.50 for a medicine that would have cost $150 without the discount scheme. His total out-of-pocket cost for the medication in the coverage gap was $40.50, comprised of a 75% copayment ($37.50) and a dispensing fee of $3. This saved him $54.50 a month compared to what he was paying before he hit the coverage gap. In the future years, as the discounts rise, recipients will find themselves in this out-of-the-ordinary circumstance more regularly.

For more information on how the coverage gap discounts apply to your drugs and how they could lower your out-of-pocket expenses during the coverage gap time, research your individual Part D plan and speak with your pharmacist or insurance provider.

Part D - shingles vaccine

Medicare Part B includes coverage for routine immunizations including the flu shot, pneumonia vaccination, and hepatitis B vaccine. When you get these immunizations from your doctor's office, Medicare will cover the whole cost. However, there is an exception to this rule: the shingles vaccination is funded by Medicare Part D.

You must be enrolled in a Medicare Part D plan, either a separate drug plan or a Medicare Advantage plan that includes drug coverage, for Medicare to pay for the shingles vaccination. Your Part D plan will establish your needed contribution toward the cost of the shingles vaccination, and you will be responsible for paying that amount.

The shingles vaccination is included in all Medicare Part D plans by law. However, depending on where you get the picture, there are several things to think about in terms of payment:

Make sure the pharmacy you visit for your vaccination is inside of your insurance's network. If it isn't, you might be responsible for paying the whole fee rather than just your standard co-pay. It's important to remember that pharmacists may get immunization licenses in any state.

If you prefer to get your shingles vaccine from your doctor's office, be sure they have the ability to electronically submit claims to your Part D plan or can connect you with a pharmacy that does. If this isn't an option, you'll have to front the money yourself and submit a reimbursement claim to your plan later.

To sum up, if you want to receive the shingles vaccination at the standard co-pay amount, you should call your Part D plan to find out which pharmacies and physicians in your region are chosen by your plan. Your vaccination coverage expectations will be met, and any unforeseen expenses will be kept to a minimum.

Medication Therapy Management benefits

Both your health and your ability to pay for medical care depend on you using just those medications for which you have a genuine need. The effects of medications on the body may be substantial, and they aren't always positive. Symptoms that weren't there before may show up if you take many medications at once for different health issues. This might lead to the need for further medicine to treat the emerging side effects. Experts in the area of safe medication always stress the need of having one's medication schedule checked up by a medical professional on a regular basis. The goal of this evaluation is to maximize the safe and effective use of drugs by identifying and carefully managing any possible interactions or side effects.

Medication therapy management (MTM) is a service provided at no cost to Medicare Part D members who meet certain criteria. The term may be cumbersome to say, but the advantage it describes is substantial, so take it into consideration if it's provided to you. Not everyone is eligible for the MTM service, so it's crucial to check with your Part D plan to see whether you qualify before deciding to join up on your own. Therefore, if your plan provides the MTM service, you should take full advantage of it to have a thorough assessment of your prescriptions performed by a healthcare expert.

Prescription medication coverage offered by Medicare Advantage HMOs and PPOs, as well as stand-alone Part D plans, must include MTM services. However, your particular plan will only extend an invitation to take use of these amenities under restricted circumstances. Plan-specific criteria may include, but are not limited to, the need for various drugs, the presence of certain chronic illnesses, or the incurrence of pharmaceutical expenses in excess of some predetermined threshold. To see whether you are eligible for the MTM services provided by your Part D plan, you should check the plan's particular eligibility conditions.

Medication therapy management (MTM) is a benefit offered by certain Medicare Part D plans, but only to those who meet certain requirements. Plan-specific variations on the following criteria are possible:

1. To qualify for Medicare Part D, you must be taking between two and eight different medications. Your strategy will lay out the precise minimum that must be met.
2. At least two or three of the following chronic illnesses must be present: diabetes, heart failure, bone disease, respiratory issues, etc. The specifics of the plan's criteria may vary in this regard.
3. If the yearly cost of drugs is more than a certain threshold, then: You and your insurance plan must spend more than a certain amount each year on prescription medications. In 2020, for instance, that amount was $4,255.

You or your designated representative (e.g., a caregiver) will be able to speak with a clinical pharmacist as part of your Part D Plan's Medication Therapy Management (MTM) program. At least once a year, this pharmacist will evaluate all of your prescriptions with you, including over-the-counter remedies, nutritional supplements, and prescription pharmaceuticals. The goal of this evaluation is to guarantee thorough drug administration.

The MTM program may also work with you to develop a pharmaceutical strategy to enhance your wellbeing.

Only your doctor has the power to make adjustments to your prescribed medications, not the MTM service. The MTM may, however, contact your physician in order to inquire about your drug history and provide advice. A complete list of your prescriptions should be provided to you and kept close at hand. You may provide this record to your primary care physician, to a specialist, or to the personnel in a hospital emergency department. Your medicines and dosages will be accurately recorded on this list.

Chapter 10
Changing Your Medicare and Medigap Coverage

Topics:

- Changing coverage during standard enrollment periods
- Switching plans at any time of the year in certain circumstances
- Separating from a plan because you or it wants out
- Figuring out whether to switch to another plan next year
- Moving to a different Medigap supplemental insurance policy

If you were faced with a plethora of alternatives when picking your original Medicare coverage, whether it was a stand-alone Part D prescription plan or a Medicare Advantage (MA) plan, switching plans may not be at the forefront of your thoughts. But it's important to know when you can switch to a different type of coverage if desired or necessary, when you can cancel your current plan (yes, Medicare has rules for that too), and whether it would be beneficial to compare plans again at the end of the year to possibly find a better deal.

Depending on your current Medicare plan and your reasons for wanting to transfer, there are a few different time periods in which you may make the transition. Key eras include the following:

1. During the annual open enrollment period (from October 15 to December 7), Medicare beneficiaries may make changes to their coverage for the next year. You may change from Original Medicare to a Medicare Advantage plan, or from one Medicare Advantage plan to another. You can also add, change, or delete a Medicare Part D prescription drug coverage at any time.
2. During the Medicare Advantage Disenrollment Period (January 1 through February 14), you may go back to Original Medicare from a Medicare Advantage plan. This option is available to you regardless of how long or short your membership in the plan has been.
3. There are times throughout the year called "special enrollment periods" when people may sign up for a plan even if they missed the deadline. If you need to make a modification outside of the typical enrollment window, you may do so during these times. Common situations include changing residence, losing health insurance via employment, and being eligible for Medicaid.

This section of the guide includes in-depth explanations of your choices for changing your Medicare coverage. It delves into the murky waters of plan cancellation and reinstatement. The end-of-year dilemma of whether to stick with your present insurance or search for something new is also discussed.

Open Enrollment or Disenrollment Switching Coverage

The two most common times of year for consumers to make changes to their coverage for the next year are open enrollment and disenrollment. The next sections provide an in-depth explanation of the many types of coverage you may change throughout various times. If you need to make a change outside of the annual enrollment period, please read on to learn about special enrollment opportunities.

Open enrollment period

If your 65th birthday is in June but you can't enroll in Medicare until October, you may be concerned about your health insurance alternatives between now and then. People who are already enrolled in Medicare are the only ones who can take advantage of open enrollment. However, if you're joining the program for the first time, you'll have your own unique enrollment window depending on your specific situation.

Every year, from October 15 and December 7, Medicare participants have a window of opportunity known as open enrollment to make adjustments to their Medicare coverage. You may change your Medicare coverage in a number of ways at this time:

1. You have the option of changing to a Medicare Advantage plan instead of Original Medicare.
2. Medicare Advantage enrollees who want to return to original Medicare may do so.
3. It is possible to switch from one Medicare Part D medication plan to another.
4. You may change Medicare Advantage plans if you don't like the coverage you're getting.
5. You may switch Medicare Advantage plans to one that covers prescription drugs if your current plan doesn't, or vice versa.
6. It is also possible to stop receiving any Medicare medication benefits at all.
7. You may also enroll in a Medicare Advantage plan or a stand-alone Part D medication plan for the first time during open enrollment if you missed the first enrollment period. When open enrollment rolls around, you may shop around for the best Medicare Part D and Medicare Advantage plan options for the next year. Beginning on October 1, information about these plans may be found on the Medicare Plan Finder website.

Even if open enrollment closes at midnight on December 7, your current coverage will remain in effect until December 31.

If you make a plan change during open enrollment, your new coverage won't kick in until the first of the year. When you enroll in a new plan, your previous plan is immediately terminated without any action on your part or notification to Medicare. However, you must notify your existing plan to discontinue coverage if you are switching from a Medicare Advantage plan to conventional Medicare or if you want to opt out of Medicare drug coverage completely.

No more action is required on your part if you just intend to maintain your existing course of action. Your current enrollment status will be carried over to the next year. It's worth noting, however, that the plan's coverage and fees could shift from one year to the next. Plan changes are discussed in further detail in the section headed "Reading your Annual Notice of Change."

Disenrollment period

Disenrollment from Medicare Advantage during the "Medicare Advantage Disenrollment Period" may be a confusing concept at first. The time frame in question is the half-month beginning on January 1 and ending on February 14. At this point, you may return to original Medicare by leaving your Medicare Advantage plan. However, during this time, you will not be able to convert from original Medicare to a Medicare Advantage plan. Some essential considerations are as follows:

- During this time, you may leave any Medicare Advantage plan you've subscribed to, regardless of how long you've been a member.
- You may switch to conventional Medicare beginning February 1 if you disenroll in January. Coverage will resume on March 1 if you cancel within the first two weeks of February.
- During this time, you may also sign up for a separate Part D prescription plan if the Medicare Advantage plan you're abandoning offers drug coverage.
- However, you will not be able to enroll in new medication coverage during this time.
- You may still buy a Medigap coverage during this time, but you won't be covered by the federal guarantees and safeguards unless certain conditions are met or your state law offers more. When you enroll in a Medicare Part D plan as a stand-alone solution, your Medicare Advantage coverage is terminated and you have access to original Medicare benefits. Unless you want to stay on your existing Medicare Advantage plan, you'll need to officially seek to be removed from it.

Advantages of Special Enrollment Periods

If you need to make a change to your Medicare coverage outside of the annual open enrollment period, you may be eligible for a special enrollment period (SEP). Generally speaking, SEPs may be cashed in at any time throughout the year, but there are strict deadlines for doing so. If you don't make a change to your plan during the open enrollment period, you will have to wait until the following year.

It's vital to keep in mind that the waiting period between plans might leave you uninsured for a significant amount of time, perhaps exposing you to late fees. In what follows, I'll go through some of the scenarios in which you could be eligible for a SEP to switch plans. I'll also cover everything you need to know to switch insurance without losing your medications or medical history.

When you can use SEPs to change plans

There are a number of situations in which a person is eligible to make adjustments to their Medicare coverage during what are called "special enrollment periods" (SEPs). However, some of the information below may also apply to your original Medicare or Medigap policy if you're considering a Medicare Advantage or Part D plan transfer. Unless otherwise indicated, "plan" may refer to either a Medicare Advantage plan or a Medicare Part D prescription plan that stands on its own.

In most cases, a special enrollment period (SEP) may be obtained with little to no effort on your part. It is the duty of the new plan you enroll in to verify your SEP eligibility; in most circumstances, all you need to do is enroll. However, you may need to file for a SEP if you feel your plan breached your contract or gave you false information during enrolling.

Contact Medicare at 800-633-4227 (TTY 877-486-2048 for those with hearing problems) to apply for a SEP in such cases. Talk to the Medicare agent about your position and why you want to transfer plans using the SEP. After doing their own investigation, Medicare will decide whether or not to approve the SEP.

You may be qualified for a variety of SEPs, not only the ones we've discussed so far. You may get a full rundown of these SEPs in the Medicare booklet "Understanding Medicare Advantage & Prescription Drug Plan Enrollment Periods." Visit www.medicare.gov/Pubs/pdf/11219-Understanding-Medicare-Part-C-D.pdf to read this helpful guide. Whether you qualify for a SEP and during what enrollment periods is explained in full.

Moving permanently outside your plan's service area

When and how you inform your current plan of your intention to transfer will determine the length of your special enrollment period (SEP). The many possibilities are as follows:

1. If you give your plan notice before you relocate, they will: Your SEP will begin one month before to your relocation and continue for an additional two months following your move month.
2. If you inform your strategy after the relocation: Two months from the day you notify the plan, your SEP will begin.
3. If you fail to inform your plan of your relocation, you will bc dropped from the plan after six months and offered a two-month special enrollment period (SEP).

If you decide to transfer plans, you may choose the effective date of your new coverage at any time. The first of the month after your enrollment in the new plan is when it will go into effect, or it may be postponed for up to three months.

Important reminders:

- Even though the firm that sponsored your old plan also provides plans in your new location, you are free to choose a new plan if better possibilities are made available to you. Moving within the same state will not allow you to switch plans if you are enrolled in a stand-alone Part D medication plan that covers the whole state.
- If you leave the coverage region of your Medicare Advantage plan, you may switch back to original Medicare without penalty. In this instance, you may also choose to buy a Medigap coverage (if you're 65 or older) that comes with all of the same government guarantees and protections as Original Medicare.

When you move into or leave a nursing home or other long-term-care facility

You may switch Medicare plans at any time throughout your stay in a nursing home, whether it's a short-term stay in a skilled nursing facility or a long-term stay in a residential home. You may need a plan that covers the long-term pharmacy used by the institution since your prescription medication needs may alter dramatically throughout these transitions.

Nursing homes, skilled nursing facilities, rehabilitation hospitals or units, long-term care hospitals, psychiatric hospitals or units, and intermediate care facilities for people with mental disabilities are all examples of the types of institutional facilities that are covered by this right to switch plans.

You have the following protections throughout your time at any of these establishments and for up to two months after you leave:

- Changing Medicare Advantage plans is something you should do.
- Make the switch from your existing Medicare Part D stand-alone plan to another one.

- Make the switch from Medicare Advantage to original Medicare and a separate Part D coverage.
- Make the switch to a Medicare Advantage plan instead of Original Medicare.
- Sign up for Medicare Part D or a Medicare Advantage plan for the first time that covers prescription drugs.

You may change plans at any time without having to request or complete a special enrollment period (SEP). It's easy; just switch to the new plan and explain your predicament. Remember to communicate your needs and preferences to ensure you have appropriate coverage during your time in the nursing home or during the transition period.

Medicare Advantage and switching to traditional Medicare

Only those who satisfy both of the following requirements are eligible to take advantage of this SEP:

1. When you first became eligible for Medicare at age 65, you probably enrolled in a Medicare Advantage (MA) plan during the first enrollment period.
2. You have just started your first year under the same MA plan.

Within the first 12 months of your MA coverage, you may switch back to original Medicare (and a separate drug plan, if necessary) provided you meet both of these criteria. Consider this first year an opportunity to "test drive" the MA plan.

In addition, you have the unalienable right to enroll in Medigap during this SEP. There is a 63-day window after the MA plan finishes during which you may apply for Medigap coverage.

During the trial term of this SEP, you may investigate and weigh your Medicare transition and coverage choices, such as regular Medicare and Medigap supplementary insurance.

Dropping Medigap policy and enroll in a Medicare Advantage for the first time

If you meet both of the requirements for this special enrollment period (SEP), you are eligible to go back to original Medicare and buy a new Medigap supplementary insurance at no additional cost to you.

1. One, you've only been part of the Medicare Advantage (MA) program for a short period of time.
2. Second, this is your first time enrolling in a Medicare health plan, and you've chosen the MA plan. Please be aware that if you have previously participated in a Medicare

health plan, regardless of whether it was Medicare Advantage or Medicare Choice, you are not eligible for this SEP.

If any of these things apply to you, your original Medigap coverage from before you enrolled in the MA plan must be restored. If you are unable to get coverage via your current insurer, you are free to shop around for a new one. With this SEP, you may leave your MA plan and return to original Medicare.

You may also utilize this SEP to enroll in a separate prescription drug plan, with coverage starting on the first of the month after your enrollment. You may take advantage of this special enrollment period by applying for a Medigap insurance up to 60 days before the end of your MA plan coverage and no later than 63 days after coverage expires.

Switching to a five-star plan

Unlike the annual open enrollment period, you don't have to wait until January 1st to switch Medicare Advantage or Part D prescription plans if one in your region has received Medicare's top five-star quality rating. Your existing plan's coverage will be terminated on the day you enroll in the five-star plan, and your new coverage will begin on the first of the month after that.

Medicare's online Plan Finder tool will tell you whether any five-star plans are offered in your region. Information regarding local five-star plans is also available by calling the Medicare assistance line at 800-633-4227 (TTY 877-486-2048).

When your plan withdraws service from your area

In each situation that qualifies for a Special Enrollment Period (SEP), you will receive a letter from Medicare, your plan, or both, providing you with important information. The letter will explain the specific circumstances that triggered the SEP, inform you about the duration of your current coverage, list alternative plans available in your area, and specify the timeframe during which you can switch to another plan.

This personalized letter serves as a notification and guide, ensuring that you are aware of your options and allowing you to make informed decisions regarding your healthcare coverage. It is important to carefully review the details provided in the letter to understand the specific rules and deadlines associated with your particular SEP.

Losing drug coverage from an employer or union, COBRA, or retiree benefits

You may qualify for a Medicare Advantage or Part D drug plan enrollment SEP if you lose or stop receiving creditable medication coverage from a current or past employer or union. If you have lost or had your creditable coverage terminated, you have two months to enroll in this SEP.

Coverage for prescription drugs that is "creditable" is defined as coverage that is at least as good as Medicare's standard coverage.

You have the option of researching and ultimately enrolling in a Medicare Advantage or Part D medication plan during this Special Enrollment Period. If you want to make sure you always have prescription medication coverage, now is the time to sign up.

Losing Medicaid or Medicare Savings Program eligibility

You may qualify for a Special Enrollment Period (SEP) to switch your Medicare Advantage or Part D prescription plan if you have been informed that you may lose Medicaid or MSP (Medicare Savings Program) coverage. You have two months from the notice date to implement the adjustments required by this SEP.

Medicaid and MSP are examples of government assistance programs that offer supplementary benefits and services to those who qualify but who may otherwise go without due to financial constraints.

During the SEP period of two months, you may evaluate your existing Medicare Advantage or Part D medication plan and make a change if you find a better one. Make the most of this registration session to lock in the coverage and perks you need.

Plan violates its contract with you

If your plan fails to deliver on its contractual obligations, such as by paying benefits on time or in accordance with Medicare's quality criteria, you may be able to quit your plan using this SEP. Medicare is the entity to whom you apply for this SEP. The SEP will begin on the day Medicare informs you that a violation has occurred. Those enrolled in a Medicare Advantage plan have the option of switching to a different plan or returning to traditional Medicare at any time. You may still take advantage of the SEP for up to 90 days after making a withdrawal. After enrolling, your new coverage will kick in on the first of the month.

Misled in joining a Medicare Advantage plan

With this SEP, you may exit a plan that you first joined due to false, misleading, or incomplete information. To be considered for this SEP, you must submit an application via Medicare. If Medicare verifies your claim, you will be allowed to switch to a different MA plan or traditional Medicare with a stand-alone Part D prescription drug coverage. (You also have the unalienable right to enroll in a Medigap supplement policy within 63 days of your plan's cancellation in this case.)

A federal employee made a mistake when processing your enrollment or disenrollment in a plan

This SEP allows you to change or cancel your Medicare Part D prescription drug coverage once an error has been made. The SEP period is two months long, beginning in the month Medicare approves it.

Making sure your records and prescriptions are transferred

When making a plan change during a SEP, it's crucial that your previous plan's data on your Part D prescription medication consumption and payments be transferred to your new plan. These documents are essential because they include key pieces of data, such as:

1. Total drug costs: The total price of all the prescription medications you've bought this year is included. It will tell you how much coverage you'll have under the new plan.
2. Total out-of-pocket expenses: These expenses are the amount you have paid for prescription drugs out of your own pocket. They count toward reaching the limit that ends the coverage gap, commonly known as the "doughnut hole."
3. Deductible payments: If your plan has a deductible, your records will show how much of the deductible you have already paid since the beginning of the year.

The transfer of the deductible amount depends on the deductible structure of your old and new plans, as well as the drug costs incurred:

- It is illegal for a new plan to demand you to pay a deductible in the same year that you have already paid one under your previous plan. The deductible is waived, and you won't have to worry about paying it again.
- If your previous plan did not need a deductible, but your new one does, you will not be covered until you have paid that deductible. If your out-of-pocket costs for prescription medications exceed the new plan's deductible, you'll have to cover the difference.
- If you haven't met the deductible in your old plan and your new plan has a deductible, the amount you pay depends on the difference between the two deductibles. If the new plan's deductible is lower, you would need to pay the remaining balance to meet the deductible. However, if the new plan has no deductible, you won't need to pay anything more, and your coverage will begin immediately.

It's important to note that "total drug costs" refer to both the amount you have personally paid and the amount your plan has paid for your drugs.

During the process of switching plans, it is advisable to review the details and coverage terms of the new plan carefully to understand how your records will be transferred and to ensure a smooth transition of your prescription drug coverage.

What happens to your unfilled refill medications when you move plans depends on the pharmacy service you use.

1. Mail-order service: If your existing mail-order pharmacy accepts your new plan, you may transfer any unused refills to your new plan. If you have questions concerning the transfer procedure, you should call your mail-order pharmacy's customer support hotline.

2. Retail pharmacy: If you use a retail pharmacy, you can continue using the same prescription only if the pharmacy is in the network of both your old and new plans. It's important to ensure that the retail pharmacy you prefer is part of the network of your new plan to avoid any disruptions in obtaining your medications. You can check with your new plan's provider directory or contact their customer service to confirm if your preferred retail pharmacy is in-network.

In both cases, it's recommended to verify the transfer process for your refill prescriptions and ensure that there will be no interruption in accessing your medications under the new plan. If you have any concerns or encounter any issues during the transfer, you can reach out to the customer service of your new plan or contact Medicare to file a complaint if necessary.

Dropping a Plan (Or Being Dropped)

Only during the open enrollment period, the disenrollment period, or the special enrollment periods described earlier in this chapter may people voluntarily drop their Medicare Advantage or Part D prescription plan. Changing from one kind of coverage to another often results in such situations. However, there are times when you may need to cut ties with one plan without immediately beginning participation in another. The plan itself may also end its contract with you under certain circumstances. Both of these cases will be explored in further depth below.

Leaving a plan on your own

You may be eligible for a special enrollment period (SEP) to leave your current Medicare Advantage or Part D medication plan without switching to a different plan if you meet one of the following criteria:

You or your spouse have begun getting health benefits from a new employer: If you or your spouse have begun receiving health benefits from a new employer, you may decline Medicare Part B or Part D prescription coverage. To achieve this, you must determine whether or not your existing Medicare Part D coverage will cause you to be ineligible for the employer's health insurance plan, and whether or not your new prescription coverage is considered creditable. Next, you should call your existing plan, provide an explanation, and ask to be dropped from coverage. Make sure that the last day of your Medicare Part D coverage coincides with the first day of your new plan.

Second, if you become qualified for military or veteran medication coverage via TRICARE or the Veterans Affairs program, you may request a Special Enrollment Period

(SEP) to leave your existing plan and enroll in the new one. Get in touch with the plan and let them know you're a TRICARE or VA beneficiary.

Third, you no longer reside within the service region of your plan because you have relocated outside the United States. Since you will not be eligible for Medicare Part D while you are outside of the country, you should contact your plan to be dropped from coverage. You are eligible for another SEP to enroll in a Part D prescription coverage plan for the two months after your permanent return to the United States.

If you desire to quit your current plan without joining another, you will not be eligible for a SEP because of #4. You often need to wait until the next open enrollment period or take advantage of the disenrollment period (for Medicare Advantage plans) to make any changes to your coverage. You are not required to enroll in another plan if you obtain a SEP to disenroll from a plan due to factors such as relocating out of the coverage region. The same holds true if you approach the conclusion of the enrollment period but decide not to reenroll (but do remember to submit a disenrollment request). It is not necessary to re-enroll in the plan if you are dropped for nonpayment of premiums.

Medicare may send you a warning letter about the danger of late fines if you elect to re-enroll in a prescription coverage plan after dropping your previous plan. However, it is essential to think about the ramifications of being without medication coverage for even a few months, in addition to the fear of late fines.

Before dropping your medication coverage without replacing it with another plan, you should carefully analyze your individual circumstances.

Getting the dropped from your current plan

In the following cases, a Medicare plan is obligated to remove you from coverage:

- You must inform the plan if you are moving permanently beyond the plan's coverage region. If they try to get in touch with you and don't hear back from you after six months, they have to remove you from the program. However, if the plan can verify that your relocation is temporary, you will keep your coverage. • If you are incarcerated, your plan must terminate your coverage. You have the right to a Special Enrollment Period (SEP) of two months after your discharge to re-enroll in a plan.
- The plan is obligated to remove you from coverage if you become ineligible for Medicare. This may happen if you were eligible because of a handicap but then recovered and no longer needed those benefits. To further complicate matters, Medicare eligibility (including Part D) will end if you pay Part A premiums but stop paying Part B premiums or notify Social Security that you no longer want this coverage. • If the plan receives evidence that you intentionally withheld or falsified information about other drug coverage you have from an employer (double-dipping),

they must disenroll you with Medicare's permission. If you are required to pay a higher-income surcharge for Part D and fail to pay it to Medicare, the plan cannot terminate your coverage until instructed to do so by Medicare. If your loved ones notify your Medicare Advantage or Part D drug plan of your death, the plan cannot terminate your coverage until they receive an official death notification from Medicare. Any premiums paid after the final day of the month after the death must be refunded by the plan.

In the following cases, your Medicare coverage may be terminated at the plan's discretion:

If your premiums are late, your coverage may be canceled. Different plans have different rules on what happens if you don't pay your premiums on time or at all. Although Medicare does not define this term precisely, it means that your actions are seriously impeding the plan's capacity to serve you and other members. Before disenrolling you for this reason, the plan is required to make every effort to remedy the problem, provide Medicare with all relevant information, and get Medicare's approval. You have the right to file an appeal, and the plan must inform you of that. For example, if you let someone else use your plan card to get services or prescription drugs, or if the information on your enrollment form was fraudulent, the plan can terminate your coverage. However, Medicare may grant you a Special Enrollment Period (SEP) to switch to another plan without losing coverage. If you are disenrolled from the plan, your participation will end on the first of the month after the plan sends you notice. Medicare must be notified of the suspected fraud and will conduct its own investigation.

Stay or Switch to Another Plan for Next Year

In the United States, November is a hectic month due to Thanksgiving and the buildup to the winter holidays. However, this is also an important moment for Medicare recipients to think about whether or not they want to keep their existing Medicare Advantage or Part D medication coverage for the next year.

From October 15th until December 7th, Medicare recipients have the option to make changes to their coverage. The new year will bring changes to your current plan's prices and benefits, and although many individuals may not think about switching plans, I urge you to do so. It is crucial to evaluate these modifications in light of competing strategies. It's possible that next year's greatest choice won't be the same as this year's, even if both were successful.

If you want to keep your existing plan for another year, you don't need to do anything; you'll be automatically re-enrolled. Though doing nothing may first seem like the most convenient choice, I urge you to give it some serious thought. It's in your best interest to compare plans and benefits before settling on one.

How and when you will be notified of changes to your Medicare Advantage or Part D medication plan is discussed below. I'll add that it's crucial to compare plans for the future year to get the best deal. Finally, I'll go through some considerations you should make if you're thinking about changing plans.

Reading Annual Notice of Change to understand plan alterations

In January, Medicare recipients often voice their frustration about unexpected cost increases. The truth is that practically every plan makes changes for the new year, which may result in substantial price and benefit changes on the first of the year. Some potential shifts include:

1. It's possible that you won't be able to enroll in this plan again the following year. This is because plans may opt not to renew their contracts with Medicare, go out of business, or even have their contracts cancelled by Medicare.
2. The sponsoring insurance company may not offer the same plan: The company behind the plan may decide not to offer it for the upcoming year.
3. Benefit design changes: The plan may modify its benefit structure, affecting coverage and costs.
4. Changes in premiums, deductibles, and co-pays: The plan may adjust the charges for premiums, deductibles, co-pays, or change the drug tiers, leading to changes in co-pays.
5. Formulary changes: The plan may alter its formulary, adding or removing drugs from the list of medications it covers.
6. Changes in drug restrictions: The plan may modify the restrictions it imposes on certain drugs, such as prior authorizations, quantity limits, or step therapy requirements.

To determine how these changes will affect you, there are specific steps to follow:

1. If your plan will not exist next year, you will receive notification from the plan or Medicare itself. In this case, you need to enroll in another plan to maintain coverage.
2. For other changes, the plan is required to send you an Annual Notice of Change (ANOC), which provides details about the modifications. This document is crucial, and it's essential to read it carefully.

Ignoring the ANOC can have consequences, as illustrated by these examples:

- Suzie didn't read her ANOC and discovered during the summer that her Part D drug plan no longer provided coverage in the coverage gap (doughnut hole). She felt deceived because she had chosen the plan based on its previous coverage. However, the ANOC she had received in the fall had warned her about the changes. Realizing her mistake, she vowed to read it in the future.

- Thomas just gave his ANOC a cursory read before he grew disturbed by the $15 annual rise in his premium. This inspired him to give the whole thing a more thorough reading. In addition, he found out that the co-pays for two of his name-brand medications will increase from $42 to $95. So, he checked up the Medicare Plan Finder on their website to see how much money he might save by switching to a different Part D medication plan for the following year. He did the math and now has the most cost-effective approach.

In summary, taking the time to review the ANOC and understanding the changes to your plan is crucial. It allows you to make informed decisions about whether to switch plans and ensure that you are prepared for any adjustments in costs and benefits for the upcoming year.

The Annual Notice of Change (ANOC) must be sent to you by the plan by September 30 of each year. The time is ideal for comparing costs and benefits for the following year to other plans. This information will also be posted on Medicare's Plan Finder website on October 1 in advance of the annual registration session. Contact your plan and ask for your ANOC if you haven't gotten it before the first week of October.

Comparing plans

I understand that comparing Medicare Advantage or Part D drug plans can feel overwhelming, but it is highly recommended by consumer advocates and myself. Here are a few reasons why shopping around is worthwhile:

1. Costs and benefits may fluctuate from year to year; this applies to your current plan as well as any other plans you may have. It's possible that the conditions of a plan that didn't work out so well for you last year may be more to your liking this year. Medicare Advantage plans may undergo changes such as price reductions, elimination of the deductible, decreased copayments, loosened medication coverage requirements, and expansion of already covered services.

2. Changes in health condition: In the previous year, your health status may have changed, necessitating a new regimen of medication or therapy. You can make sure that your current health insurance plan is the best fit for your requirements by comparing it to others.

3. Lowest premium and drug coverage: If you are not presently taking any medications and have selected the Part D plan with the lowest price, it is still worthwhile to compare the premiums of the various plans for the future year.

4. Peace of mind: By comparing plans and confirming that your current plan remains the best option for you, you can have the peace of mind that you have made an informed decision and are getting the most suitable coverage.

Remember, the open enrollment period provides a valuable opportunity to review and potentially switch plans.

The ease with which one may use the Medicare website's annual plan comparison tool is an additional argument in favor of doing so. It may take just a few minutes if you know the process and what to look for to decide whether your current plan is still the best choice or if another plan provides superior coverage.

By regularly comparing plans, you'll become more adept at navigating the Plan Finder tool and understanding the information provided. This can save you time and effort in the long run, making the decision-making process more efficient.

Factors influencing your decision

If you have reached the point of considering one or two alternative plans to your current coverage, it's important to carefully evaluate your options before making a final decision.

Exceptions from your current plan

Find out whether your current plan's exceptions will transfer over into the following year if they have covered a medicine that is not on its formulary or waived a limitation on any of your prescriptions based on your doctor's advice. Depending on the plan, you may need to reapply for an exemption in the next year. The exclusions policy of the plan is detailed in the plan's documentation. If this is not made clear, you should get in touch with the plan and ask for specifics in writing.

Allowing exceptions to be carried over from one year to the next may be a huge time saver and may be a decisive factor in whether or not to continue with your current plan. If, on the other hand, your plan does not permit exclusions to be carried over, you have nothing to lose by investigating other plans. However, it is important to evaluate the limitations of any other programs you may be contemplating. Some or all of the medications you use regularly may fall under this category.

Making an educated choice about whether to stick with your current plan or move to a new one requires knowing how your exceptions will be handled in the next year. You can better meet your pharmaceutical requirements if you clarify this information and evaluate the limitations of different options.

Switching to a Medicare Advantage

Comparing the prescription coverage, medical expenses, and advantages of the Medicare Advantage plan with those of regular Medicare and a Part D drug plan is essential before making the transition.

If you have a Medigap policy, you should think about it alongside your prescription medication coverage and healthcare expenditures. Medicare Advantage plans provide a 12-month "trial period" for new enrollees who forgo Medigap coverage in favor of them. You have the option to go back to original Medicare and enroll in a Medigap coverage with the same provider at the same rates during this trial period. If you decide that the Medicare Advantage plan is not right for you, you may switch back to your original Medigap policy during the special enrollment period.

After the trial period ends, if you elect to return to standard Medicare and buy a new Medigap coverage, you may not be entitled to the same government guarantees and protections that were included in your old policy. Therefore, the premium for the new plan might be higher than the premium for the old plan.

As an example, consider the following: After turning 65, Erica originally registered in regular Medicare and then added a Medigap coverage to her healthcare portfolio. She had Medigap coverage until 2017, when she opted to switch to a Medicare Advantage plan instead. Several months later, she recognized that she had made a mistake. Given that she had been enrolled in the Medicare Advantage plan for less than a year and that this was her first and only Medicare Advantage plan, she was instantly eligible to switch back to regular Medicare and resume her previous Medigap coverage.

Before making the jump to a Medicare Advantage plan, it's important to weigh the impact on your Medigap coverage. You can better meet your healthcare requirements by making a decision after considering all of your alternatives and the length of the trial period.

Changing your Medigap Policy

If you currently have a Medigap policy and are considering whether to switch to another policy, it's important to understand the factors involved and make an informed decision. While purchasing the best Medigap policy you can afford initially is often recommended to avoid complications, there may be valid reasons for wanting to change your policy over time. Here are some common situations that might prompt a desire to switch:

1. You're paying for benefits you don't really need: As your healthcare needs change, you may find that your current Medigap policy includes benefits that are no longer necessary or relevant to your situation. In this case, it may be beneficial to switch to a policy that better aligns with your current needs, potentially saving you money on premiums.

2. You now need a policy with more benefits: On the other hand, your healthcare needs may have evolved, requiring additional coverage that your current Medigap policy does not provide. If you find yourself in this situation, switching to a policy with more comprehensive coverage may be advantageous.

3. You're not satisfied with your current insurance company: If you're dissatisfied with the customer service, claims handling, or overall experience provided by the insurance company that issues your current Medigap policy, you may want to explore other options. Switching to a policy offered by a different insurance company could lead to better service and satisfaction.
4. Another policy or company may offer cost savings: Over time, insurance companies may adjust their pricing and premiums for Medigap policies. By comparing the available options, you may find that switching to a different policy or insurance company could result in cost savings without compromising the coverage you need.

When considering a switch in Medigap policies, it's crucial to carefully review and compare the benefits, costs, and terms of the new policy you are considering. Additionally, be aware of any restrictions or waiting periods that may apply when switching Medigap policies. It is advisable to consult with a knowledgeable insurance professional or Medicare counselor who can provide personalized guidance based on your specific circumstances.

Remember, making an informed decision and avoiding costly mistakes is essential when it comes to choosing or switching Medigap policies.

It's important to address a few misconceptions regarding Medigap insurance to clarify how it works and alleviate any concerns about losing coverage:

1. Although Medicare Parts A and B both have yearly open enrollment periods, there is no such thing for Medigap coverage. It is common to refer to the first six months following Medicare Part B enrollment as "Medigap open enrollment." You may buy a Medigap insurance now without worrying about being turned down for coverage due to your health, as long as you meet the policy's health requirements.
2. Guaranteed renewal of your Medigap policy: Once you have purchased a Medigap policy, you have the right to renew it every year without any action required on your part. This guarantee is contingent on providing accurate information on your application and continuing to pay the premiums.
3. When you travel across the nation seeking medical attention from doctors and hospitals that accept Medicare, your Medigap coverage will follow you. Getting a new Medigap coverage is usually unnecessary if you relocate. It is possible that you may need to buy a new Medigap coverage if you move out of the service region covered by your current Medicare SELECT policy.

It's important to understand these facts about Medigap insurance to avoid unnecessary confusion or concerns about losing coverage. Remember to review your Medigap policy annually and ensure that it continues to meet your healthcare needs.

Consequences of switching Medigap policies

It's important to note that federal law does not grant you an absolute right to switch from one Medigap policy to another with the same full federal guarantees as when you initially purchased your policy. The ability to switch Medigap policies and the ease of doing so may vary depending on your location and the specific requirements set by your state or the insurance companies.

Different states have varying regulations regarding switching Medigap policies, and some states may have more consumer-friendly requirements in place. It's essential to understand the rules and regulations specific to your state when considering switching Medigap policies.

You will need to convince either your current insurer or a new Medigap insurer to offer you a new policy if you want to switch your coverage. This may include looking into your medical history, underwriting criteria, and the plans offered by various insurers.

Even while it's feasible to transfer Medigap insurance, you should know that you may not be afforded the same federal protections and guarantees as you were when you first acquired your coverage.

Before embarking on the process of switching your Medigap policy, it's important to understand the provisions under federal law and the additional protections offered by certain states. Here are some key points to consider:

1. Pre-existing Conditions: Under federal law, an insurer cannot exclude coverage for pre-existing medical conditions or impose waiting periods for coverage if your current Medigap policy has been in effect for six months or longer.
2. Temporary Denial of Coverage: The insurer can temporarily deny coverage for benefits in the new policy that are not included in your current policy. However, this temporary denial cannot exceed six months after the new policy takes effect.
3. Premiums Based on Age and Health: The insurer may require you to pay higher premiums based on your current age and state of health.
4. Insurer's Discretion: The insurer has the right to refuse to sell you a new Medigap policy.

It's important to note that some states offer additional protections and opportunities to switch Medigap policies without considering your current health status or pre-existing medical conditions. For example:

- In the 30 days after your birthday each year, you may modify your existing Medigap coverage to one with the same or less benefits, or transfer insurers, in the states of California and Oregon.

- You may change to a different Medigap coverage in Maine at any time, whether it's one with the same or less benefits.
- In Missouri, you have the option of switching insurers for your Medigap coverage within 60 days after the policy's anniversary date..

Get in touch with or check out the website of your state's insurance department to learn the ins and outs of Medigap coverage in your area. You may find the address and phone number of your state's insurance department on the website of the National Association of Insurance Commissioners (NAIC) (www.naic.org/state_web_map.htm).

Exploring a change of Medigap coverage

To compare different Medigap policies and switch to a new policy, you can follow these steps:

1. Utilize Medicare's website to compare the benefits offered by different Medigap policies. The website will provide details on available standardized policies labeled A, B, D, G, K, L, M, and N in your area.
2. Contact your current insurance company and inform them of your intention to switch to another Medigap policy. They will guide you through the process and may ask you to complete an application form and answer health-related questions.
3. If your current insurer declines your request or if you prefer to switch to another company, create a list of other insurers in your area that offer Medigap policies.
4. Be mindful of how each insurance is rated. Insurers who employ community rating or issue-age rating systems are worth keeping in mind if your existing insurance has an acquired age rating (where rates grow with age). Insurance policies rated using these methods often have cheaper premiums.
5. Contact the insurers on your list and inquire whether they offer the specific Medigap policy you have chosen. If they do, request a quote for the premium.
6. Evaluate the advantages and disadvantages of switching to a new policy versus retaining your current one. Consider factors such as the benefits provided, the reputation of the insurer, the premium cost, and your personal health needs.

By following these steps, you can effectively compare Medigap policies, contact insurers, and make an informed decision about switching to a new policy or staying with your current one.

Your right to a 30-day free look

To qualify for a new Medigap coverage, you must give up your old one. However, the cancellation may be postponed for up to 30 days after the start of your new policy, as required by federal legislation. This time, often known as a "free look," is a trial period and a helpful consumer protection mechanism. You'll have a chance to give the new policy some thought and make sure it meets your needs throughout this period. You are free to revoke your acceptance of the new policy and keep your current one if you change your mind. It's crucial to remember that throughout this 30-day window, you'll be responsible for paying premiums on both plans.

Chapter 11
Medicare Misconceptions

Topics:

- Identifying potential enrolling difficulties to prevent
- How to choose a Medicare supplement coverage (Medigap) and a Part D medication plan
- The ability to access resources for cost cutting

Most new Medicare enrollees likely won't have much experience navigating the system. It's not quite a minefield, but there are several hazards that may be disastrous if not approached with caution.

If you want to save money and be happy with Medicare, it's important to avoid making some of the most frequent errors people make. People who were uninformed of the enrollment criteria ended up either going without coverage for long stretches of time or paying higher rates for the rest of their lives, given what I've heard.

Medicare and Social Security aren't compelled to advise people who are about to turn 65 about their Medicare enrollment options at this time. Therefore, many individuals make poor choices with potentially disastrous financial outcomes because they lack information. It is hoped that this situation will improve so that everyone may get the help they need to enroll in Medicare and understand the program's requirements.

The BENES Act was brought into Congress to remedy the inadequate counseling of those interested in enrolling in Medicare. If this bill passes, people would start getting reminders a few months before they turn 65. The message would explain how to enroll, provide detailed instructions depending on the recipient's personal situation, and offer a phone number to call with any queries.

The BENES Act is a major advance in ensuring that people are protected against potential enrolling hazards. However, Congress has yet to approve the bill as of this writing.

This chapter provides a streamlined checklist of the top 10 Medicare errors to help you avoid making them. It's a helpful resource for making sure you're prepared for the registration process and know what you're doing.

You don't need to Reach Full Retirement Age before Signing Up

Medicare enrollment and the commencement of Social Security retirement benefits used to occur concurrently for many people. The following information, however, is relevant in light of the new circumstances:

The age at which one may get their full Social Security benefit has increased. This age ranges from 66 to 67 for most individuals nowadays, depending on when they were born. If you or your spouse do not have other health insurance via work, Medicare enrollment before age 65 is essential to avoid late fines.

It's important to remember that you may sign up for Medicare at any time, not only when you become eligible to receive Social Security payments. Both programs have their own application and enrollment deadlines. To prevent late fees and coverage gaps, it is crucial to familiarize oneself with Medicare's enrollment guidelines and to join at the proper time.

Don't Assume You Don't Qualify for Medicare

Understanding the eligibility requirements and enrollment timelines for Medicare is crucial to ensure a smooth transition and avoid potential penalties or gaps in coverage. While earning at least 40 credits through payroll taxes guarantees premium-free Part A benefits (hospital coverage) after joining Medicare, no work credits are necessary for Part B (medical services) and Part D (prescription drug coverage). To qualify for Part B and Part D, individuals aged 65 or older need to pay the monthly premiums, regardless of their work history.

However, if you lack 40 credits at age 65 and delay signing up for Part B until earning them, there may be a waiting period for coverage and potential permanent late penalties. By understanding these intricacies, you can make informed decisions and ensure timely enrollment without incurring unnecessary costs or delays.

It's Crucial to Enroll in Part B When You Should

Medicare enrollment at the right time is critical for avoiding penalties. Inaction on your part might result in non-payment or late fees.

Delay in coverage: if you miss the first registration period, you may join up between January 1 and March 31 of the following year, during the general enrollment period. Coverage won't start until July 1 if you enroll during this time, however.

Fees for being late: If you wait more than 12 months to sign up for Medicare Part B, the monthly premiums for the following years will increase by 10%.

If you or your spouse actively work for an employer that offers health insurance and that company has 20 or more employees, you are exempt from this requirement. If this is the case, you may put off signing up for Part B until your current employment expires without any penalties.

Sign up within your seven-month initial enrollment period, which usually begins three months before the month you turn 65, to avoid these possible hazards.

You Need Part B

Part B of Medicare enrollment is voluntary; however, it's important to know that coverage from sources like retiree benefits and COBRA coverage do not count as "active" employment and therefore do not shield you from penalties for enrolling late in Part B.

Retirement Perks: Carefully examining your retirement plan's compatibility with Medicare is essential. When you retire, Medicare often takes over as your main insurance, and the retiree plan only kicks in for a handful of extras. Part B enrollment is mandatory, and missing the deadline might leave you unprotected.

If you lose your job and qualify for COBRA, you may keep your health insurance coverage from your previous employer for up to 18 months at full monthly cost. If you are eligible for Medicare Part B and have not enrolled by the time you turn 65 or within eight months of your employment ending, you may be subject to late enrollment penalties.

Part D – You still need Prescription Drugs

Since it is hard to know what medical expenses you may incur in the future, it is prudent to pay your Part D premiums even if you are not presently in need of prescriptions. An unforeseen sickness or accident might leave you in need of costly medicine, such as cancer treatments that can cost several thousand dollars monthly.

Like other types of insurance, Part D will kick in when you need it to pay medical expenses. You can't put off signing up until your drug needs are dire, however. Unless you have "creditable" prescription coverage from sources like retiree benefits, which Medicare considers similar to Part D, you risk accruing permanent late penalties added to your Part D premiums if you delay enrolling in Part D.

Not having access to necessary medication is the more severe consequence of skipping Part D enrollment. You will need to wait until the next open enrollment period to enroll in a Part D plan if you do not enroll within your first eligibility period and have no other qualifying prescription drug coverage. The registration period lasts from the 15th of October through the 7th of December each year, and coverage begins on January 1st. Choosing a plan with the cheapest premium can get you covered while keeping your costs down.

Picking the wrong Part D Drug Plan for the Wrong Reasons

Do not choose a Part D plan based on erroneous criteria such the premium amount, your acquaintance with the plan's name, or the plan selected by your spouse or friend. Instead, you should think about the particular medications you're already taking. various Part D plans cover various medicines and have different co-pay requirements for the same prescription. Your actual out-of-pocket costs are determined less by your premiums than by your co-pays.

You can choose the best Medicare Part D plan for your needs by comparing the plans' premiums and the medications they cover. Medicare's online Plan Finder might be a useful resource here.

Confusion of Enrollment Periods

The Medicare open enrollment period, which runs from October 15th to December 7th each year, is for current Medicare beneficiaries only who desire to make changes to their coverage for the next year.

Medicare first-time enrollees may choose from a few distinct enrollment windows. The first enrollment period, which lasts for seven months and normally begins when you turn 65, is one possibility. On the other hand, there are also limited-time opportunities to enroll. You or your spouse may be eligible for a special enrollment period if you already have health insurance via your employment. There are additional special enrollment periods for those who are eligible for Medicare because of a disability, who are temporarily residing outside the United States, or who are legal immigrants.

There are potential repercussions if you miss your chance to enroll in Medicare during your personal registration period and instead wait until the general open enrollment period (October 15 to December 7). You may lose coverage or be subject to permanent late fines if you miss your individual deadline.

Being unable to purchase Medigap with Full Protection in time

Traditional Medicare has certain out-of-pocket costs that may be covered by purchasing Medigap supplementary insurance. Buying Medigap when you are 65 or older is crucial if you want to take advantage of all the government safeguards available to you. Insurance companies cannot refuse to cover you or increase your premiums because of your health if you purchase a Medigap insurance during the first six months after enrolling in Part B, or under certain other conditions. However, outside of these periods, insurers may be able to do so unless you happen to live in a state with more protective laws.

A Medigap policy may not be eligible for federal protections if purchased more than six months after Medicare Part B enrollment if the policyholder continued to be covered by their employer's insurance after retirement. You may still qualify for government protections by purchasing a Medigap coverage during the first six months after turning 65 if you registered in Part B before reaching 65 due to a disability..

Not Reading Your Annual Change Notice

If you have a Medicare Advantage plan (HMO or PPO) or a Medicare Part D prescription drug coverage, you will get a significant document in the mail each September. This paper details the next year's pricing and benefits modifications for the plan. It alerts you to changes in your premiums and drug price tiers that may raise your out-of-pocket costs for prescription drugs.

This notice contains important information that will help you evaluate your current plan and the options open to you in the future year. There is a step-by-step guide available in (Part D medication plans) and (for Medicare Advantage plans) that you may use to compare plans and see if there is a better alternative for you during the open enrollment period, which runs from October 15 to December 7. You have the option to switch plans for the next year if you discover one that better suits your needs.

If you continue with a plan that has raised its prices for the new year and you failed to receive this notification, you may be in for some unpleasant surprises on January 1. Make the most of the open enrollment time and make sure you have the best plan possible by staying informed.

Being Aware of Your Potential Eligibility for Cost-Reduction Assistance

If you're facing financial constraints and find it challenging to afford the expenses associated with Medicare, there are three programs you should explore to potentially reduce those costs, provided you meet the eligibility criteria:

1. Medicaid: People with extremely low incomes may get health insurance at a much-reduced cost via this state-run program. If you are eligible, Medicare will be your main insurance, and Medicaid will be your secondary insurance, paying for Medicare's share of your medical costs and maybe covering things that Medicare doesn't.

2. Medicare Savings Programs: Administered by the state, these programs assist individuals with incomes below the state-set limits by paying for Part B premiums and, in some cases, other expenses related to Medicare.

3. Extra Help: This federal program offers low-cost or discounted Part D prescription drug coverage for individuals with incomes and savings below a certain threshold.

Investigating these options may help you get the healthcare services and drugs you need without breaking the bank on Medicare.

It is suggested that you contact your state's SHIP to find out whether you qualify for the programs outlined. SHIP provides free advice and help with Medicare and Medicaid issues. You may find the toll-free number for your SHIP in Appendix A, which also lists several other Medicare-related services and organizations.

Getting in touch with your local SHIP can provide you with personalized guidance and support in navigating the application process and determining your eligibility for programs that can help reduce your Medicare expenses.

Checkoff List

- Medicare – Medicare Advantage
- Prescription Plan
- Dental – Vision Insurance
- Long Term Care
- Disability Insurance
- Cancer – Heart Attack – Stroke Insurance
- Home Health Care Insurance
- Accident Insurance
- Life Insurance
- Pension Plan – "Start your own."
- 401K/403B Roll-over – Management
- Will/Trust
- Health Care Directives
- Living Will
- Medical Power of Attorney
- Financial Power of Attorney
- Beneficiary Forms
- Estate Tax

This is a short list of what you need to talk about and have in your safe.

Personal Information, Family History, & Financial Information

- Birth certificate
- Adoption papers
- Marriage License
- Prenuptial agreement
- Divorce documentation
- Immigration or citizenship documents
- Social Security cards – Login information
- Military DD-214 service record
- Driver's License – copy
- Health Insurance cards – copy
- Passport

Short list of copies that you need to have in your safe

Who to Contact list

- Who to contact after emergencies
- Contact information for close friends and neighbors
- Medical & health information, list of current medications
- Blood type
- Doctors/physicians
- Medical history
- Allergies
- Immunization records
- Employer details
- School and day care contacts if children are attending
- Pets – veterinary information
- Financial Advisor
- Attorney
- Estate Attorney
- Insurance Agent
- Banker
- Accountant
- Trust Officer
- Executor
- Guardian
- Power of attorney for financial
- Power of attorney for health care
- Power of attorney for physician & other relevant medical professionals

Short list of what you need to know and have in your safe

Made in the USA
Monee, IL
02 November 2026

67384815R00103